PLEASURE GUIDE

LINZI DREW'S
PLEASURE GUIDE

Outrageous Sex and How to Have It

Linzi Drew

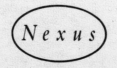

First published in Great Britain in 1992 by
Nexus
338 Ladbroke Grove
London W10 5AH

ISBN 0 352 32837 1

Typeset by Avocet Typesetters, Bicester, Oxon
Printed and bound in Great Britain by
Cox & Wyman Ltd, Reading, Berks

Contents

Introduction

I truly believe that the one most important sexual organ is the brain. In other words, no matter what the length or girth of your lover's penis, or the tightness or wetness of your vagina, sex is all about attitude. More specifically, an attitude that releases us from all sorts of sexual guilt, one that enables each and every one of us to allow our head to be perfectly in tune with our body's responses — which in turn can reward us with exquisite sexual pleasure. We must make a stand and claim our sexual liberty, and we must do that by getting on and enjoying our new-found sexual freedom. But these days, when we women are seeking our independence, you may ask: 'Why should any woman want to become the perfect lover? Doesn't that just imply that she intends to become some sort of sex toy?' The point is that every woman has the enormous potential of having enjoyable, ecstatic sex. In fact, women are in the privileged position of being able to have more fun with sex than men! Both men and women have the right to enjoy wonderful sexual pleasures, and by learning about our bodies and loving them we can reach a new peak of sexual fulfilment.

The first step towards getting to know and love our bodies is exploration. With regard to men this statement would seem to be somewhat amusing and obvious, as most males discover their penis and the joys of masturbation even before they can walk! But time spent caressing your cock and touching other parts of your body will naturally be arousing and will ultimately result in discovering new ways to pleasure yourself, which in turn will enable you to teach your lover what pleases you the most. Try gripping your cock in different ways, handling it firmly or perhaps very gently. Use both hands, maybe, or keep one hand free to play with your balls, slide a finger into your anus or squeeze your nipples. Experiment with oils and lotions and enjoy your body to the full.

All this may seem very elementary, but for women this is often not the case. Because our pleasure potential is tucked away, we must seek to find. Set aside some time to be alone and then take off all your clothes. Examine your breasts to see which form of stroking and caressing gives you the most pleasure. Try sitting on the floor, perhaps, in front of a mirror, your legs wide open, and take a good look at your pussy. Spread your lips open, examine your clitoris, and then slide a finger inside. You know, it's amazing to think that we possess such a fascinating sexual organ and yet there are still many women who have never really taken a good close look at it! How can you ever explain to your partner what turns you on if you're not sure yourself? Men aren't mindreaders, you know!

Here we come across another sexual stumbling block: openly discussing sex with your partner, be the conversation about a slightly bizarre fantasy or just what specific sex act really arouses you. Building and maintaining a satisfying, loving sexual relationship is not always easy, but it is definitely worth striving for. We must inform our lover when a certain type of caress is particularly stimulating, just as we must when one tickles or is too rough. For instance, when I give oral sex to my lover, I like to look into his eyes to see exactly what's going on in his head, but it also helps a great deal if he can talk me through my technique. One rule I like to keep for my sexual pleasures is that making love is not about performing, it is about *being*. Trying to perform interferes immensely with sensual pleasure. And what brings us more pleasure than letting go, and thinking and breathing positive sexual energies, leading us to orgasm?

How important is an orgasm for a woman? We all know that if a man can't achieve orgasm he's usually the butt of jokes and packed off to a sex therapist, but no such thing happens with women. Many women go through their entire life without ever experiencing the intense pleasure of orgasm, and that I find a great shame. From their very first sexual encounter and throughout marriage, some stumble along without any real clue about the joys of making love. But don't doubt it: the pleasure potential is there and with this pleasure guide I'm going to help you to find it.

Please don't get the idea that sex is such a serious subject. It's not. It's special, it's emotional, yet it should be light-hearted and fun. A couple who barely exchange two words whilst in the throes of fornication must be doing something wrong! Go on, admit it — there's plenty of times when you can't concentrate on your sensations because you have cramp, or times when you want to take a rest or crack a joke! When you're both approaching fever pitch, I'm sure the conversation will turn to something far more colourful!

And girls, don't be afraid to take the initiative — for goodness' sake, if you're horny, let him know! Something as unique and special as sex really is a labour of love. In this book, I advocate that you practise, not theorise. When it comes to making love, practice is much more fun than theory anyway!

With the pace of today, it is important that we set aside time for sex. Create the perfect environment, whether it's in the bedroom, the back seat of your car, or in the bath. This planning of lust can be a tremendous turn-on, a form of extended foreplay. Perhaps you could indulge in mutually agreed sex games, with only touching and no actual penetration for an allotted period of time. When you actually make love, all that anticipation will be an added delight. Foreplay can be a tremendous turn-on.

Experimenting with sex toys and masturbation is not only acceptable but a pleasure to be savoured. After all, it's the first step towards finding out what really arouses you. And mutual masturbation can add an extra dimension to your sex life, not to mention the enormous role that it can play in safe sex.

Finding Mr or Ms Right these days is not quite as simple as it was when I was taking my first tentative sexual steps. Unfortunately AIDS is something we can no longer ignore and brush under the carpet, ignorantly saying, 'It's a homosexual disease'. AIDS can be transmitted when blood, semen or vaginal love juices enter the body during sexual intercourse, so these days we need to find our partner and stick with them. Or, if we want to wander, then we wander well stocked with good-quality condoms. But if you're fortunate enough to have found your perfect partner, for goodness' sake hold on to them with both hands! Even if you've had sex with the same person more times than you can count, there's every reason that it should get better and better, nor worse! I know a sexual relationship can lose spontaneity and urgency after the first few months or so, but then is the time to begin to work at it. Experiment with perfecting the art of oral sex; make love in as many unusual places as you can think of; discuss your fantasies and, if you are both in agreement, act them out (assuming they're legal!). Girls – dress up for sex. Find out exactly what turns him on. If you know it will stimulate him to see you dressed in thigh-high boots and crotchless panties, then surprise him when the moment is right. You'll be the one at the receiving end of the frenzied fire in his loins! And I suggest that if kinky capers get you in the mood, have a go!

I'm sure this book will make you want to have a go! I've even included a selection of sexercises that should help keep you toned up and in tiptop condition for all the energetic sexual activity that you're sure to be having. My motto is 'Practice makes perfect'! My pleasure guide is based on all my experiences as a woman, and on the many letters I have received whilst working as editor of *Penthouse* magazine, and, of course, on what I have learned talking intimately with my friends and lovers. You may believe that because I was employed by a magazine featuring sexually explicit photographs of women I am exploiting my own sex, 'letting the side down'. But personally I can see nothing whatsoever wrong in glorifying and glamorising the female form, and obviously the men and women who've opened up to me and contributed to this book have no argument with my views. Thank goodness the powers that be have recently seen fit to allow us women an equivalent of *Penthouse* – *For Women*. No stiff dicks, but I suppose it's a start!

My main focus is on sexual pleasure as a thing of great beauty, not as something professional spoilsports insinuate is wrong and dirty. You must decide as a couple what you want to experience sexually. For instance, if your man wants you to tie him up and allow him to wear your frilly knickers and the idea appeals to you, then why the hell not (as long as they fit!)? Equally, if you fancy a *menage à trois* with your bloke

11

and his best friend, and you think you can all handle it, what has it got to do with anyone else?

I sincerely hope that you will enjoy this book and that it will in some way assist you in coming to terms with your sexuality. Your course in perfect pleasure-giving and receiving starts here. I must admit that it's going to take a fair bit of application and effort, but what better way to spend your free time than learning how to stimulate your clitoris or penis with your lover's fingers, tongue, penis, pussy . . ? The list of ways to attain the peak of sexual pleasure is enormous, so it's your duty to make the time to try them all! I hope that when you've finished reading, you will have realised all the passion, sensuality and tenderness to which you are entitled, and be good and ready to seek out your perfect partner, grab them with both hands, and please each other beyond your wildest dreams!

LINZI DREW, 1992

1

Am I Good in Bed?

How can we possibly know if we're sexually adequate in bed? And of course, even if we do, we all want to be much better than just adequate anyway! When it comes to making love, my watchword is *relax*. Not so much that you're in danger of nodding off, but just enough to lose all your inhibitions and enjoy the excitement that is lovemaking. I think probably one of the most upsetting insults ever is to be told: 'You're a lousy fuck!' Thankfully I've never been accused of this, not because I haven't been guilty of it, but perhaps because I'm always eager to learn and that eagerness always seems to shine through.

First and foremost, we should come to terms with the male and female sex organs. If you're scared to take a good look at your lover's penis or vagina, you're not going to be terribly arousing at oral sex! Just the same, your partner may wish to pay a great deal of attention to your sex, either with their tongue or their fingers, and will perhaps want to admire you at close proximity. Where's the fun if this makes one of you hot to trot, but embarrasses the other no end? And what if the thought of oral sex actually terrifies you? I suspect that giving is always the more daunting prospect. I remember vividly the first time I sucked a cock. I really didn't have a clue what to do, but quite

13

unashamedly I asked for directions! And that is what we must do to become the perfect lover. It's not that difficult, but sometimes we don't want to discuss sexual techniques for fear of hurting our lover's feelings. We must discuss them in a caring and adult manner. Who knows, your partner too may not be overawed with your sexual performance, and if you ignore the issue you will never achieve your true sexual potential as a couple.

I was sitting down with a girlfriend of mine and we were indulging in a little sex talk. Jane, a country girl from Swindon, told me: 'My sex life has improved over the last few weeks and it's because, for once, I wasn't too shy to make the first move. I've been dating my boyfriend Thomas for almost six months now. We'd made love two or three times a week and it was generally pretty good. Always with him on top of me, which does excite me, but somehow or other I found that I had to play with myself as well to reach a climax.

'Then the other night we'd been out to a party and a few glasses of red wine had made me very randy. When we got home I was feeling so sexy that I stripped out of my clothes almost immediately and we started kissing. Without even thinking about it, I told him I wanted to fuck him. I wanted him to lie down and I wanted to impale myself on his cock. Thomas loved the idea and couldn't get into position quick enough. That first time riding on top of him, feeling his cock much deeper inside me — well, I was so turned on, I climaxed three or four times.'

It's fabulous that Jane could lose her inhibitions with the help of a couple of glasses of wine, and could discover new joys in their lovemaking. It doesn't always work out so happily, though. Belinda, a PR consultant from Manchester, told me: 'After being married to John for three years our marriage broke up. Before getting wed, I'd only been with two other men and neither of them had really turned me on. Once I was married my sex life was what I supposed to be usual. Nice in parts, but often pretty boring. John would make love to me quite regularly and seemed to me to be enjoying himself. He always made the first move and I always went along with it, never thinking to suggest any variation to his routine.

'I only wish I had, because a few months ago the rumours started filtering through, John stopped making love to me, and I found out he was having an affair with a girl at the office. Even though I was thoroughly demoralised, I tried to make an effort, by concentrating more on my appearance and dressing in sexy lingerie. I was desperate to cling on to a man I really do love, but all to no avail. We had a final showdown and he told me he was leaving me because he'd fallen for this girl at work. I was devastated, especially when he told me it was all because I was such a "cold fish" in bed!'

It's an unfortunate truth that Belinda is not alone in her misery. Over the years, I have received many such letters with sorry tales of losing a loved one just because of boredom and lack of sexual satisfaction. In fact, whilst working as editor of *Penthouse* magazine, I was often treated as an agony aunt by frustrated males unhappy with their sex lives. Amazingly they were able to put down on paper and send off intimate details of their problems and disappointments to a complete stranger, yet they were unable to discuss these same problems with their loved ones!

This letter that I was sent is typical. Tim of South London wrote: 'I've been with my present girlfriend for almost a year now. I love her very much and we intend to get married in the next year or so. She's good-

15

looking, caring and very intelligent. Our sex life is quite good, but I know it could be so much better! My girlfriend Caroline is so shy about sex. She rarely lets me look at her body, is embarrassed when I suggest something new and if I ask if I can watch her masturbate or put forward the idea of her dressing up in something sexy, she blushes like crazy and tells me I'm kinky. Maybe I am! But I just want to experiment. I don't want to do anything to upset or hurt her, I just want both of us to have as much fun as possible with sex!'

Naturally! I think Tim sounds like the type of guy who will work it all out in the end, just as this lady from Belgium who wrote to me did. Marie Jeanne had lost a husband, but after some time alone, she suddenly seemed to find the sexual freedom she so much desired: 'I am forty-five years old and have had four children during my twenty-three-year marriage to a very possessive husband. When my husband died, I married a man who is seven years younger than I am. With him, I learned for the first time in my life that there is much more to sex than I had in my previous marriage. My husband is much more sexually orientated and allows me to dress sexily. All the time he makes me believe that I can still seduce men. With him I feel reborn! Two times now I have made a threesome with him and a friend of his, and I have to admit that I loved every minute of it. One of them had a long thin cock, on which I sank with a very hot and juicy fanny. My husband sat near us in the grass (we did it in the garden) and played with his own tool, as he was very excited with the show that I was putting on with his friend. Near orgasm, he hurried to me, put his cock in my mouth, and shot a full load of semen in it which I swallowed very eagerly, while his friend shot his load deep into my pussy. At the same time I climaxed like

16

never before. Those and other things I would like to do every day!'

Another positive attitude from a sexual woman, showing the exact qualities needed to stop the rot long before it sets in, comes from a conversation I had with a friend, a model called Tara who comes from Buckinghamshire.

I have had a good bit of sexual experience and I really do enjoy sex, but when I met my new boyfriend Simon, I really wanted to hold on to him. You'd love him, Linzi, all the girls in the village fancy him; he's tall, good-looking and successful. I thought if I could really wow him in bed, then he's going to stick around. Not to mention the fact that I'll have some fantastic fucks into the bargain!

The first night we made love was just perfect. We went to the cinema and sat in the back row holding hands for a while. When I thought the time was right, I reached over and laid the flat of my hand on the bulge in his trousers. Keeping my eyes on the screen, I cupped his prick and balls very gently squeezing them. Soon I could hear his breathing become laboured and his erection growing. I was dressed exactly for this moment, in a shortish dress, complete with stockings and suspenders. Simon was aware that I was spreading my legs for him. He knew exactly the game I was playing and reached over and started to stroke me. He let out a gasp of pleasure as his hands met with my silky stocking tops. That was just the beginning. We missed the end of the movie and hurried home to my flat to get down to some serious sex.

We started off in the shower. He soaped by

breasts and I leaned back into him. I wriggled my creamy bottom against his thighs and felt his erection gently probing between my buttocks like a warm wand. Soon his hand slipped between my thighs, fingering me gently and opening me up. After that we moved on into the bedroom and things got even better!

Now that is what I call planning an evening of lovemaking! Tara seemed to have it all worked out. In this busy day and age, planning and making time for lovemaking is essential. I always think that a pleasant way to learn about your lover's body is by taking a shower together. There's nothing more sensuous than washing and soaping each other in a hot steamy shower. Use just the tips of your fingers, working in gentle circular movements, paying particular attention to the back of the neck, the small of the back and the nipples. Press your bodies together and then explore each other's mouths. Go on, really kiss. The union of lips is a very underrated pastime in many maritial beds. Kissing is one of the first steps that sets the brain into an arousal mode. Personally, I think that if he can't turn you on by kissing you, he's not your Mr Right!

Now, girls, after you've parted your lips and teeth and are exploring his mouth with your tongue, you will be eager for him to stroke your breasts. We women are all unique and the type of caress that may drive you crazy would perhaps do nothing at all for me. So tell him exactly what you like. You may well appreciate a butterfly touch or delight in quite vigorous squeezing. If he hurts you, you must tell him at once. Remember, he wants to make love to you, not cause you pain. When he finds a particularly stimulating caress, tell him exactly how it feels. When you want him to use his

18

mouth, gently push his head towards your breasts. Hold his head and urge him on as he goes to work on you.

By this time I suspect that something very big, stiff and throbbing will be poking you in the midriff! Gently take hold of him and grasp his cock near the base, with your fingers together on one side of his shaft, your thumb on the other. Ask him if he wants you to take a firmer grip on him and let him direct you as you slide your hand up and down his shaft, perhaps cupping his balls with your other hand.

Now might be as good a time as any to make mad passionate love in your shower cubicle with the hot water splashing continuously on your bodies. Or, on the other hand, you may want to prolong the anticipation by adjourning to the lounge, the hallway or the kitchen. But let's face it, the bedroom is the most convenient venue for lovemaking, and for leisurely, varied sex it is definitely the place to be. But that doesn't mean that because you're doing it in bed it's lights off and a quick few thrusts before the male rolls off the female. Oh no! On top of the covers in a warm, dimly lit boudoir is the perfect place to make love for hours on end.

Gina, a striptease artiste from Norfolk, told me how she and her husband Eric play in their bedroom.

'Eric and I have a great time sexually. We like to do it in all sorts of places, but to be honest there's no place better than on our bed. We have this enormous four-poster which is just perfect if I'm feeling a little kinky and want Eric to tie my hands and feet to the bedstead. The bed's size also makes it great for changing position. We start off screwing in one position and after a great deal of thrashing around, Eric starts climaxing in about our fifth or sixth chosen fucking position.'

Gary, an accountant from Oxfordshire, revealed: 'When I meet a girl and I really want to make love to her for the first time, I try to save it for the bedroom. It's all very well having a grope in the car on the way home, but on my king-size waterbed I can really put everything into it. Trying to be romantic and bring her to orgasm with my tongue on the backseat of my Ford Sierra does have its limitations. I like to see her fully naked in my lowly lit bedroom, watch her strip and then explore every inch of her with my tongue and fingers before fucking her for as long as we both desire — and the bedroom is the perfect place for it!'

Wendy, a nurse from London, confessed to me: 'I love playing around with sex, but my favourite place when it comes to making love is in my bed and in the missionary position. But that doesn't make me a boring sexual partner, I can assure you! The other evening my boyfriend Michael spent about two hours playing with me. I writhed around on my bed for ages while he smothered me in oil and gave me a wonderfully sexy massage. Then he shaved off all my pubic hair and licked my cunt until I climaxed more times than I can count, before fucking me with a ripe, peeled banana. Naturally he made sure I was well and truly fucked after that little lot! I was on my back in the missionary position and we both had a great time!'

Making love at home in the comfort of your own bedroom certainly has a lot going for it. OK, sometimes the thrill of slipping a fumbling hand inside frilly panties that are getting wetter by the minute, in the cramped confines of the back seat of a car, is unbeatable; but as Wendy knows only too well, there's more than one way of building up to an incredible fuck! Aside from shaven havens, oils and lotions, and banana splits, a very simple way to excite both yourself and your lover is to indulge in a little striptease. I've been

20

a professional stripper in my time, and where better to utilise the slow, sensual build-up of striptease than in your bedroom?

Linzi is in her boudoir where soft music, low lights and a huge brass bed set the scene. Her man sits or lies in front of her. She dresses in a slinky evening dress that buttons down the front, and high-heeled shoes. She sways to the music and rubs her hands slowly over her body. She turns away from her man and lifts her skirt, flashing her stocking tops and pushing out her bottom to show off its roundness. She smooths her hands over her buttocks, digging her long red nails into her silk panties.

Turning, Linzi faces her lover, starting to unbutton her dress, slipping it gently from her shoulders, revealing her flame-red brassière, then lowering it to expose matching panties. Flinging the dress to one side, she stands rigid: hands on hips, shoulders back, breasts thrust out. She starts to play with her breasts through her bra, letting her fingers creep inside to excite her nipples. Unclipping her front-fastening bra, she lets her breasts spring free and sucks a finger in her mouth, tracing a line to a nipple before circling a wet trail around it. Meanwhile, the other hand slides inside her panties and strokes to please herself. Now she turns away again, stands with her legs almost together and bends forward a little, easing her panties down, exhibiting her bottom and exposing a peek of her pink vulva. When her panties are around her ankles, she slowly turns to offer herself totally.

(1991 *Sex Maniac's Bible*)

Unfortunately I know that not all men and women are confident enough with themselves and their bodies to go through that type of scenario. But you must always

21

remember that your lover is with you because they find you attractive, and one thing I've learnt that many men and women do find very exciting is a sensual and uninhibited partner. So why not try it, when the mood and the time is right?

Choosing the right time and moment is also very critical. Deborah, an old school chum from Bristol, revealed to me: 'I nearly fell out with my boyfriend Sam because I was doing the right things at the wrong times. Sam commutes every day to London and gets home quite late in the evening sometimes. I spend my days alone and generally get very horny by the time he gets in from work. Usually the moment he walked in the door, I'd be all over him: kissing him, sucking his dick, and then demanding that he fuck me. Sam always went along with it and I thought everything was hunky-dory. But the other night when I took his dick out, he stopped me, just sat me down and explained that some nights he just wanted to sit down, enjoy a drink, read the newspaper, completely relax and then think about fucking!'

So just being keen isn't always the answer to being good in bed. One thing is for sure: very few of us are so good sexually that we can't improve our techniques, and even more importantly, none of us is so bad that there's no hope of improvement! It's not possible to suddenly change from a shy, retiring mouse to an insatiable tiger or tigress overnight. No, you need help from this book and, of course, from an understanding lover. Remember at all times that the most important skill you can learn is that of communicating sexually with your chosen partner. One other vital ingredient is the ability to feel confident with yourself and the desire for sexual variety within your relationship. Below I have listed ten handy tips that I think will help you ladies feel good, and these in turn will keep the men in your life feeling happy and horny. Ten quite basic ideas for finding new sexual pleasure that could make a world of difference to your lovemaking . . .

LINZI'S TOP TEN TIPS FOR THE LADIES

1. Keep yourself in good condition by taking regular exercise. There's a series of easy-to-follow exercises further on in this book that can help keep you in tiptop condition.
2. Although I do advocate that you spend plenty of time in bed, do make sure you get *some* beauty sleep while you're there!
3. Take long baths and spoil yourself with a rich bath oil. Masturbating in the bath is one of the most relaxing, enjoyable pastimes I know.
4. Keep your skin soft and moist by using plenty of body lotion. Ask a friend to help rub it all over. That can be fun!
5. Make sure you dab your favourite perfume in all the right places, as you never know when your lover may not be able to resist you!
6. If you can have a weekly body massage, it really alleviates stress and helps you relax. Follow it up with an invigorating body rub, which tones muscles and loosens all dead skin cells, leaving you feeling totally refreshed.
7. One thing that always makes me feel sexy is just a little alcohol. A few glasses of white wine or a couple of bucks fizzes are perfect to loosen you up and get you in the mood.
8. Pamper yourself. Visit your local beauty salon and have a facial, a manicure and pedicure.
9. Take particular pride in your appearance. Treat yourself to a new lipstick or a pair of cherry-red silk panties. Glossy painted lips and the feel of

smooth silk will make your randy and will probably drive your man crazy!
10. Make your bedroom into a sexual boudoir. Prepare the bed, fill the room with fresh flowers, buy some candles, dim the lights and put on your favourite music.

By now you should be feeling very confident, looking and feeling great, and eager to try out some of my other ideas!

LINZI'S LIST OF SEX GAMES

1. Read and reread my technique for striptease, and surprise your partner by putting on those new undies and having a go!
2. Plan an evening of sex. Perhaps start off by dressing up and going out to a restaurant, where you can turn each other on by eating asparagus decadently with your fingers and tongues, then play with your partner under the table. No doubt you'll end up fucking as soon as you leave the restaurant and get into the car! Even better if it's a taxi! Then bring your evening to a climatic conclusion by making leisurely love at home.
3. I've stressed the convenience of making love at home in bed, but why not try it in other places around the house? Ever tried the kitchen, or enjoyed a good session over the dining-room table? Make out a timetable and sexually work your way around your home!
4. If you trust him, girls, ask him to tie you up. If the idea worries you, just ask him to tie your legs and leave your hands free. If you fancy being the dominant one, tell him that you are going to tie him up. When he's helpless, tease him mercilessly

24

until neither of you can stand it any longer and you sit astride him and fuck him. This position is very satisfying, not only for the thrill it gives you by being on top, but also because it is one position that achieves very deep penetration.

5. Plan a session of oral sex. No genital penetration must take place. Spend the entire day or evening talking and playing with each other, revealing exactly what turns you on. Perhaps dabble with deep throating or sample the 69 position. Personally I don't find the 69 position very satisfactory, as I like to give my full attention to whatever it is I'm sucking, but experiment to find out exactly what gives you and your partner fullest satisfaction.

6. I've already mentioned massage as a great way for relieving tension, but it's also a great way to get horny. Play around with massaging your lover's body with aromatic oils. I've devoted an entire chapter to sexual massage in this book, so you've no excuse!

7. If the weather is good, go out and find a quiet secluded place to have sex out of doors. There's nothing better than the suspense of wondering if you're being watched, and the wind in your hair and your knickers as you succumb to a deliciously decadent knee-trembler under a big tree or down a dark alley.

8. Get hold of some erotica: either watch a sexy movie together or read real-life letters from my letters file in *Men's Letters* magazine. I'm a great believer in talking explicitly about sex. Don't be embarrassed – it's good dirty fun!

9. Speaking of talking dirty: choose your moment carefully, and then give your lover a sexy phone call. Describe to them exactly what you're wearing

and tell them how you are pleasing yourself just thinking of them. By the time you meet up later, are you going to get it!

10. Girls take the initiative and do something really kinky! Surprise him by shaving off all your pubic hair, dressing up in crotchless rubber knickers to cook his tea, telling him you'd like to make love to another woman, or asking him to slide a peeled cucumber into your pussy. Use your imagination, that's the key. I'm sure you'll think of something bizarre that will give you both a good time!

Let's hope some of those handy, horny tips get you in the right mood! You know, physically and mentally lovemaking can be one of the most sensational experiences of your life, and it's one hell of a way to while away a lazy Sunday afternoon! So do be prepared to learn, and do be ready to indulge in those funny little sex games that may seem a little embarrassing at first, but which go on to awaken a craving for delicious sexual pleasures. Remember, practice makes perfect and if you keep on talking dirty, massaging his cock with oils, her pussy with lotions, and experimenting with every different sexual position imaginable, you're going to have a lot of fun and become very proficient in bed. Perhaps even a legend in your own bedroom!

LET'S RECAP!

- 'I think one of the most upsetting insults ever is to told: 'You're a lousy fuck!' Thankfully I've never been accused of this, not because I haven't been guilty of it, but perhaps because I'm always eager to learn, and that quality seems to shine through!'

- 'I remember vividly the first time I sucked a cock. I really didn't have a clue what to do, but quite unashamedly asked for directions.'

- 'Without even thinking about it, I told him I wanted to fuck him. I wanted him to lie down and I wanted to impale myself on his cock.'

- 'Near orgasm he hurried to me, put his cock in my mouth and shot a full load of semen in it which I swallowed eagerly, while his friend shot his load deep into my pussy. At the same time I climaxed like never before. These and other things I would like to do every day!'

- But that doesn't mean because you're doing it in bed that it's lights off and a quick few thrusts before the male rolls off the female.

- 'Trying to be romantic and bring her to orgasm with my tongue on the back seat of my Ford Sierra does have its limitations!'

2

Sex Toys and Masturbation

What costs nothing, doesn't hurt a soul and feels absolutely fantastic? Playing with yourself, masturbating, wanking, call it what you will! From a very early age, if Mummy doesn't scold us for touching ourselves; we explore that pleasurable area between our legs and for the first time experience the warm rush of sexual excitement. Naturally we have no idea why it feels so good, but as we get older we learn the techniques that suit us and give us the most satisfying reward.

Masturbation is the major step for learning about what pleases us sexually. You guys have an organ so designed that I would imagine it's difficult to leave alone in boyhood, but we girls don't have it quite so easy. We don't have this phallic addition dangling between our legs; we have to go much further and explore the treasures hidden within.

The first masturbatory sensation that I can bring to mind is trapping a pillow tightly between my legs and literally riding it to orgasm. Even now it still works for me, but I must confess I prefer to use a man's taut muscled leg whenever one is available! Doctors and Nurses is a game that I remember playing quite enthusiastically, both with the boy next door and with three or four girlfriends. I don't recall what my views were on this type of activity at the time, but I suspect it was something I thought I shouldn't be doing but which was definitely fun!

One thing that absolutely astounds me about masturbating is that in this day and age it is still a taboo subject. People *still* say it makes you go blind, and the like. Both men and women are actually bashful about admitting they indulge, and we even insult people by labelling them a wanker or a tosser! If you were to walk down the street and call out: 'Hey wanker!', every honest person should turn around and say, 'Who, me?' Mind you, I'm not suggesting for a moment you try this experiment!

Thankfully this isn't the case with everyone. In fact, I know many people with whom I can discuss the delights of self-satisfaction – men and women who feel totally relaxed with the concept of sexually arousing themselves. Bringing myself to orgasm is, for me, a way to relieve stress and relax totally, and it is a pastime that can be enjoyed by each and every one of us without guilt or embarrassment. And girls, we have so many wonderful sex toys to assist us. As a rule men seem to pore over erotica, and need only this and one or both of their hands to bring them instant sunshine. We're very different, and, as luck would have it, there are numerous sex aids on the market to bring us wonderful hedonistic pleasure. I asked a group of my female friends about their masturbating techniques.

Karen, a hairdresser from Berkshire, told me: 'I masturbate a lot. I was at the health club with a mate, and we both had a half-hour session on the sunbeds. When we came out she said to me how boring it was to lie there for thirty minutes. So I told her she should play with herself. I feel you can masturbate anywhere you feel comfortable, whenever you want to, just do it. I couldn't do without it. I remember there have been times when I've been driving home and I'd be that horny that I'd actually plan it out — you know, premeditated masturbation on the way home from work! I'd plan my route so that I'd know exactly where I would stop to finger myself. Sometimes I think I'm sick, but then I think it's fun and I'm not hurting anybody, so why not?'

Carrie, a twenty-four-year-old, happily married mother of two, spoke candidly of her collection of sex aids: 'I've got so many sex toys that if I walk into a sex shop, unless they've had a new delivery in recently, I have every toy in there! Anal beads are my favourite at the moment. I'll put four or five pairs up my arse and two in my pussy. I'll try anything. My favourite vibrator is one that you plug in. It's just the worst thing when you're almost there and your batteries run low. I'll tell you something funny that happened a few months ago. I had this vibrator that you attach different bits on to the end. The one that I really loved wanking with had this soft cushion-type attachment. So there I was laid back on my bed, my legs spread, rubbing my clit like crazy with this wonderful little vibrating cushion, and I must have got so carried away, it fell off. I just had to have my cushion to finish me off, so I got some Superglue to stick it back on, but the Superglue cap fell off and stuck my vibrator to the bed. I was going crazy!'

Deirdre, a model from Holland, has a very unusual sex toy: 'I use my razor, you know, those wet-and-dry razors. I use that instead of one of those big, ugly dildos, which to me are a total turn-off and make a terrible noise. You just take the wet-and-dry and take the top off. Get rid of the blade of course, and then I just work it up and down against my clitoris. If I want to have an orgasm real quick it's perfect, and you can travel with it too!'

Personally I prefer my fingers with a handy bottle of baby oil, but each to their own! Lisa from the east end of London seemed to me slightly more traditional in her preferences: 'I love playing with myself and do it whenever I've got the time. I suppose I masturbate once or twice a day, in addition to getting fucked regularly, I must add. I own two vibrators and a dildo. One of my vibrators is the silver bullet type and very small, so I can keep it in my handbag and use it whenever I can slip off somewhere private to do so. I've got this big dildo as well that is black and absolutely fucking enormous. Probably about twelve inches. When I wank myself with that I just shove it all the way in and leave it buzzing inside me while I squeeze my clit. I like to wank with that when I'm feeling really dirty, but usually I just use my fingers, cover my cunt in lots of baby oil and then just finger myself. I like to take ages to make myself come. You know, build up to it a few times and just about when I'm on the brink, I stop for a moment and then go for the big build-up again. By the time I finally come, it's so intense it just seems to go on and on!'

Sharon, who works in TV, explained to me in a little more detail the euphoria that can be attained from her favourite sex toys − love balls: 'I've named them anal beads. There's five little balls on a string and I like to stick them up my arse, then finger myself with one hand. Then just as I'm about to have an orgasm, I pull the balls out one at a time, but all the way out. It's incredible, it really prolongs my orgasm.'

I did get round to talking to some male friends about how they like to wank. Micky is single and approaching his fortieth birthday, and has come up with the rather apt title of 'solo flying' for wanking. He told me: 'As well as having sex regularly, I love solo flying. I suppose on average I do it about three times a day. When I sleep alone I always wake up with an erection. A quick wank with one hand, dreaming of the lady in my life or whilst gazing at some sexy girl in a magazine, puts me in the right mood for the day. I don't understand the stigma about it. It feels good, it's free and I for one love it!'

My sentiments entirely! And just a few of these snippets of conversation enlighten us to the liberated attitudes and the various ways that these individuals pleasure themselves. I have a healthy sex life, but I also love to wank whenever time allows and, like Karen, when bronzing my body under a tanning bed, I always let my fingers do the walking. Like Lisa I carry a pocket-size vibrator in my handbag for convenient surreptitious wanks. Sneaking off someplace to play with myself makes it all the more fun. And like Micky I think there's few better ways to start the day than with a wank — except perhaps with a fuck!

Aside from catching a few minutes during a busy day to enjoy an orgasm or two, I like to plan a leisurely few hours alone specifically to play with myself. And there are so many ways to make the whole scenario ecstatic. My favourite music is a must, as is a thoroughly comfortable location — I generally choose my bedroom. I like to dress up in sexy lingerie, so that I can enjoy the pleasure of firstly stroking myself through silky panties, then pulling them off to one side before I really get down to business. I am very aroused by the visual aspect of sex, so I position a mirror at the end of my brass bed. Through the brass rails I like to watch my golden bullet vibrator plunging in and out of my pussy, and I savour that buzzing sound as the whole of my cunt comes alive. Or alternatively I enjoy my fingers, drenched in baby oil, stroking my greasy clit until it swells to twice its normal size and feels like it's on fire!

Talking of using music to add to the stimulating

sensation reminds me of an amusing letter I once received. Frank, a widower from Bath, wrote to me to describe his pleasure: 'I love wanking to music. I find nothing more exciting than putting on my favourite classical music and wanking in time to the stroking of violins, booming of the bass drums and clashing of cymbals. I use my dick as a baton, stroking its entire length, building up as the music reaches a crescendo. My favourite tune at the moment is "Rule Brittania"!'

For people like Frank, wanking is probably their entire sex life. There's no shame in enjoying your own body as he obviously does.

Ignorant bigots might have a right good giggle at the thought of some lonely, elderly man stroking his baton to 'Rule Brittania'. But why not? It's his body reaching that mind-numbing crescendo! Dogmatists would exhibit their usual intolerant attitude and cast ridicule on a chap that gets his kicks from plunging his dick into a blow-up rubber doll. But why the hell shouldn't he? It's his dick pumping away inside that plastic paradise. Don't mock what you haven't tried!

Of course, masturbation is often practised by single people who for some reason are without a partner, and by men and women who are separated from their partners for periods of time. For instance, I could say that almost all of the guys in Her Majesty's Armed Forces are wankers, but that doesn't mean they won't fight the good fight! I should know exactly what they get up to; thousands of them write their dirty letters to me describing in explicit detail how pleasurable wanking can be. But believe me, I don't need to be convinced! Here's a few samples of the kind of horny, yet amusing correspondence, starting with a letter from some jolly Jack Tars:

'I expect you get loads of letters from bored,

frustrated sailors. Well, we are at present on exercise for four weeks with no contact with the outside world. As most of us are chefs, we just love to eat food off our partners' bodies, but we can't think of anything better than to lick yoghurt off your super-duper nipples and lovehole.

'We wonder what you're up to at this moment in time – 30 May, 9.17 p.m.? We've had a vote and the majority say you're getting it doggy fashion with another cock in your mouth. Were we right? Probably not exactly spot on, but the mere thought of it had us all in a wanking frenzy!'

The next letter from the 'Desert Rats' was short and straight to the point: 'At the moment there are five of us in a tent with a picture of you. About five minutes ago, all of us wanked at the same time and spunked all over your photo. Could you please send us another?'

How could a girl refuse such a plea? Now to conclude these mucky masturbation masterpieces, a squaddie in Turkey wrote: 'Serving in Turkey is hard work and hot work and what makes it bad is that I am bursting for a good fuck. My only contact with sex at the moment is the magazines that my wife has been sending out to keep me on the boil for a bloody good sex session when I get home. I've been ogling some pictures of you. Your ample tits and your sweet cunt always manage to give me a good lob-on. How I would love to slide my cock deep inside your pussy whilst I explore your mouth with my tongue. I long to lick at your pussy. Oh, what a magic taste a good cunt is, and you have one hell of a tasty-looking slit.

'Anyway to the point of my letter. Would you take pity on a sex-starved squaddie and send me a signed photograph to lust over? Perhaps to make it extra special you could see your way to signing it, kissing it and maybe rubbing that sweet pussy of yours all over it? Go on, please!'

Somewhat cheeky, maybe, but erotic photographs obviously help these guys keep their spirits and their peckers up!

Naturally I am not advocating that masturbation can replace love, affection and a fulfilling sex life, something I think we all want and need. But it can be an immensely pleasurable pursuit, a welcome addition to a good sex life or, in the absence of any sex life to speak of, a way to keep you going till better times come along!

Aside from giving lonely or disunited people some form of a sex life, masturbation can also provide a valuable way to help keep fraught marriages together. Sadly it's often the case that one half of a partnership is disinterested in sex from time to time, not infrequently when there are other problems and stresses within the marriage. All of us experience peaks and troughs of desire. Everyone has a baseline sexuality which has to do with age, upbringing and their general attitude to sex. And most people are more sexual when they're feeling good about themselves than they are when they're feeling bad. This ego-libido correction is usually stronger in males than in females, so if the problem is only that of a temporary abstinence, masturbation can more often than not see the other half of the partnership through the barren times!

John, an elderly, retired friend of mine from the midlands, has been married for over forty years, and for the last five years his wife has shown little enthusiasm for sex. John, on the other hand, has an avid interest. He revealed:

The other night I went to bed dreaming I was rubbing baby oil all over a TV actress. I'll mention no names! The naughty things I think of in the privacy of my own bedroom would astound you. Most of my respectable friends have stopped having sex. One said he'd rather have a corned-beef sandwich and a half of shandy!

Now my wooing days are long since gone, I don't want to get hung up and frustrated. I find the titillation of magazines recharges my batteries. I am Ever Ready! I like to get my rocks off in a passionate way and vary my routine. I admit I enjoy watching porno movies. The women really put the men through their paces. Some people say that too much fucking saps your body and wanking affects your brainpower. What a lot of twaddle! A healthy sex life keeps you young and vital. And every now and then the missus catches me at it and seems vaguely interested!

I know I joke about my pal and his corned-beef sandwich. Of course sex sometimes drops off when you've been married a long time. I now get my rocks off by reading magazines and watching blue movies. My wife understands that, because to us both, friendship counts a lot in our relationship. But it still is wonderful to look back on our early married times.

So far in this chapter we've been discussing masturbation as a solitary pleasure. But mutual masturbation is a wonderful way to learn what excites your partner, and is perfect to indulge in with someone you've just met − both of you can peak sexually, yet still be responsible and practise safe sex. It's also one hell of a way to spend a lazy afternoon! I know from experience that men enjoy watching a woman masturbate, and for me that is a great turn-on. I have one boyfriend who told me the other day that all he needs to do to get me in the mood for a great fuck is for him to ask me to let him watch me play with my pussy. He was right − spot on, in fact − but funnily enough I hadn't even realised how much it excited me! I too love to watch a man wank himself off. Sometimes I can hardly decide where to focus my eyes. Should I stare at his engorged prick or the expression on his face?

Now if you feel exactly as I do that wanking with a partner is perfectly acceptable and immensely pleasing, please keep on at it. On the other hand, if you or your lover can't quite come to terms with it, do relax and give it a try. Put aside a whole evening to explore. Make your bedroom or lounge as comfortable and intimate as possible. Dim the lights just a little, or perhaps buy some candles for that special ambiance. Select some relaxing music and start off by undressing each other. To feel confident, girls, make sure you are dressed in your sexiest undies. You may want to experiment by using just your fingers and hands, but I suggest that, before this delightful planned evening of masturbation, you take a trip to a sex shop and purchase one or two aids to play around with. Perhaps he might start off with a vibrator or a dildo for her; and maybe, girls, you could get him some sexually explicit magazines or some of those exciting anal beads for retrieval just at the precise moment of his ejaculation!

The whole idea is to relax and not be embarrassed about arousing each other manually and allowing the other to watch while we stimulate ourself to orgasm. Let your partner see what excites you, and show them how to stroke you in the most effective, exciting way. That is the key to learning. One of my favourite sex games is to bring myself to orgasm with my lover watching closely; just as I'm about to come, he slips his cock right into my orgasmic pussy. Perhaps I'll try pulling beads out of my arse at the same time. Wow! Am I going to have a prolonged orgasm!

Because this chapter is all about masturbation I have featured lots of letters from my days as editor of *Penthouse*. Whilst editing and appearing nude in a magazine of that genre, I was, as you can imagine, inundated with letters regarding wanking. One that I found particularly sexy focused on solitary masturbation and led on to a couple enjoying mutual masturbation; it was from Dave in Essex. Dave wrote:

I just had to write to you about an incident that was potentially the most embarrassing of my life, but which turned out to be one of the most enjoyable. It was at the start of this recent hot weather. An urge came upon me to go out and buy *Penthouse*. I hadn't bought one for a few months and was looking forward to a leisurely evening alone with my *Penthouse* (while my girlfriend Lisa was out giving private Spanish lessons) and to a good wank. Well, I'd forgotten how good the magazine is. I went to my bedroom, stripped to my boxer shorts and wanked twice over the letters pages alone. Boy, those letters were hot. But that was just the start. Where do you find all those beautiful girls? I went rock hard at the sight of each and every one of them. I shot my load again, imagining that those stunningly sexy women were naked in my bedroom, thickly coating their mouths in bright red lipstick, then slowly sucking me off — one of my favourite fantasies — before putting my throbbing, lipstick-stained knob inside their glistening tight pussies.

By now it was getting dark and I had been lost in my own fantasy world for more than an hour.

My penis was purple and sensitive and I was pretty knackered. But I forgot my tiredness when I turned the page and saw the first of a series of shots of you, Linzi — the sexiest selection of erotic photos I've ever had the pleasure of seeing. I came just by looking at your tits. Despite the heat in my bedroom I shivered with pleasure at the thought of what my tongue and tool could do for your exquisite pussy.

Anyway, to get to what could have been the embarrassing bit: I was masturbating over your picture so fiercely that I didn't hear the front door open, my girlfriend come in, climb the stairs and enter the bedroom. I'm sure she could hear the sounds and thought I had a woman in there with me.

At first she was open-mouthed. Then before I could say anything, she pulled up her skirt, pulled down her pants and told me to carry on masturbating, but looking at her pussy and not yours!

Lisa joined me on the bed and at first I carried on wanking, staring at her pussy lips that were getting juicier and juicier as she frigged herself. She told me not to touch her as she spread her legs, faced me and stuck two fingers inside. Her pussy was bright pink and bulging now as I watched her finger-fuck herself until she came. Then she allowed me to suck on her fingers and drink her come. Gripping my swollen dick I told her I wanted to bend her over and fuck her like a dog. I thought I would explode if she wouldn't let me inside her soon. Playing with her boyish tits, she chastised me and informed me that I'd probably been coming all evening and now it was her turn. Relenting slightly, she allowed me to wank her to her second climax, and then she got really generous. She spread open her pussy lips and let me lick her to her third orgasm, before demanding that I fuck her doggy-style to her fourth orgasm of the evening! I think I still came out on top.

Anyway, now Lisa insists on buying me *Penthouse* each month, and every Monday night after her Spanish lesson we play the same kind of game. I wank at home alone in the bedroom, anticipating all that fun to come when she gets home and catches me red-handed!

Lisa and Dave make masturbation a prelude to some sucking and fucking. Sounds like fun to me! I think there's been enough said in this chapter to convince any reluctant wankers that it's fun and free, and that there's no shame in it. I'd conclude by telling you that writing about it has made me feel so randy that I've got to dash off and have a wank, but that kind of frivolous remark gets printed only in men's magazines — besides, typing one-handed is a doddle! But I will nevertheless bring this chapter to a conclusion by recommending some fascinating sex aids.

- A Glow-In-The-Dark Vibrator, available from Knutz, 1 Russell Street, London WC2.
- Anal Love Beads — enormous black rubber ones on a rubber string. Available mail order from the Rob Gallery, Weteringsschans 253, 1017 XJ, Amsterdam.
- Strap-On Clitoris Vibrator: 'Judy's Butterfly' is available from Yago Holdings, Unit 18, Roman Way, Coleshill Ind. Estate, Coleshill, Birmingham B46 1RL.

- Vibrator with foreskin which slides back and forth — also from Yago Holdings.
- A copy of the video *Linzi Drew's Striptacular* — one hour dedicated to erotic striptease. And *Members Only*, the adult video magazine presented by and featuring me! Both are as raunchy as the laws of this land will allow and are available mail order from Brittania, and from high street video shops.

LET'S RECAP!

- 'The first masturbatory sensation that I can bring to mind is trapping a pillow tightly between my legs and literally riding it to orgasm. Even now it still works for me, but I must confess I prefer to use a man's taut muscled leg whenever one is available.'
- 'Through the brass rails I like to watch my golden bullet vibrator plunging in and out of my pussy and savour that buzzing sound as the whole of my cunt comes alive.'
- 'I use my dick as a baton, stroking its entire length, building up as the music reaches a crescendo. My favourite tune at the moment is 'Rule Brittania'!'
- 'Oh, what a magic taste a good cunt is, and you have one hell of a tasty-looking slit!'
- 'Most of my respectable friends have stopped having sex. One said he'd rather have a corned-beef sandwich and a half of shandy!'
- 'One of my favourite sex games is to bring myself to orgasm with my lover viewing at close proximity, and just as I'm about to come, he slips his cock right into my orgasmic pussy.'

3

The Art of Kissing

My dictionary's definition of a kiss is a 'touch or caress with the lips; a touch with the lips as an expression of love or desire, or as a greeting'. But of course a kiss is so much more. It is perhaps the most familiar and widely practised physical expression in our society today. It is possible to make a list of the numerous ways in which we use this caress with our lips, from footballers planting an enormous great smacker on the mouths of colleagues after they've slammed the ball into the back of the net, to the false affections awarded to casual aquaintances – the pressing of dry, closed mouths to proffered cheeks at social gatherings; from warm, welcoming kisses that accompany hugs and cuddles dished out to close friends and families to the kisses used in religious ceremonies. But of course the kiss we shall be exploring in this chapter is the sexual kiss.

Naturally the kiss plays a very important role in our sexual behaviour and strict guidelines are always drawn between social and sexual kissing. For instance, a man instinctively knows when a woman will accept a kiss on the cheek or the mouth. If it is to be planted on the mouth, then he has to decide whether or not to part his lips or use his tongue. The insertion of his tongue into a woman's open mouth can be very symbolic and reflects the act of lovemaking. Often a couple can adopt the exciting rhythm of fucking. And if the female partner takes the initiative with her tongue, then symbolically she is offering penetration to him. Think about it, girls. How many times have you enjoyed a lengthy tongue-tussle and the minute your fella decides to slip his hands down your panties, it's time to go home? You'll get yourself a reputation as a prickteaser, you know! Actually, it's my opinion that when a man's concentrating on sticking his tongue halfway down your throat and his trembling hands are wriggling all over your quivering body, he isn't thinking symbolically! I frequently relish this kind of kissing, and it has to be said that I'm the kind of girl who's always happy to take the lead. In fact, I think that first tentative kiss as it builds in passion is one of the most stimulating sexual experiences there is. I suppose my theory is that if the first, tender kiss is good, there's a lot more to come!

We can call upon the poets to offer up their imaginative, flowery explanation of the sexual kiss. Coleridge called a kiss 'nectar breathing', while Shakespeare referred to it as 'a seal of love'. The Roman poet Martial described it at some length: 'A kiss is the fragrance of balsam extracted from aromatic trees; the ripe odour yielded by the teeming saffron; the perfume of fruits mellowing in their winter buds; the flowery meadows in the summer; amber warmed by the hand of a girl; a bouquet of flowers that attracts the bees'.

Heady stuff! I'm pretty sure that Essex Man or the like won't be whispering those kind of sweet nothings when he fancies a snog in the back of his motor! Having never been considered much of a poet myself, my idea of a sexual kiss isn't quite as romantic. That doesn't mean I don't consider it exhilarating, sensual and exciting. Personally, a sexual kiss is the commencement of foreplay, the first pleasurable moment when the union of lips begins the arousal process.

The mouth, lips and tongue, like all the other mucous membranes of the human body, are erogenous zones. The tongue especially is full of sensitive nerves that send signals to the genitals, signals that seem to give me that first twitch, that first sexual stirring. Test your oral sensitivity by practising these simple experiments:

- Relax and position your lips comfortably. Make sure they are thoroughly dry, and with the tip of your forefinger gently slide your finger firstly along your lower lip and then along your top lip. Notice how smoothly your finger moves along its surface. Hopefully you will feel a slight tingling sensation.
- Now try the same exercise wet. As Bon Jovi inform us with their raunchy album title, it's 'slippery when wet'. And they're damn right! Stick your finger in your mouth and suck on it. Let your tongue rest upon it, but no tongue exercises for the moment. Don't worry — we're steadily building up to that! Now that your finger is nice and wet, lick your lips until they too are thoroughly lubricated. Use your finger once again to stroke both top and bottom lips. This time you'll find the sensation feels completely different. It slips rather than slides. The sexual glow this exercise awards me is slightly more acute. I suppose this is because wetness and sexual arousal gel so nicely together.
- Finally you're ready to slide that forefinger right into your mouth. Just the tip at first and lick it with your tongue. Move your finger about and let your tongue move in a circle around it. Now insert your finger further into your mouth so that your tongue

now concentrates on your knuckle and beyond. You will notice the mobility of your tongue and the different textures of its upper and lower sides. And, ladies, this can also be used as a method to practise deep-throating, but I shall be coming to that in a couple of chapters from now. This last exercise is the most arousing of the three and is not often indulged in as a solitary sport. Men offer their forefinger to their partner's mouth. Naturally this symbolises the acceptance of their pricks between their lover's eager lips. And we all know how much you guys enjoy having your dick sucked! Don't worry, fellas; as I've already said, we shall be exploring fellatio at great length very soon. Of course, I am fully aware that it's far more fun practising these kinds of games with a partner, but take it from me, these little self-stimulation exercises can be a very useful way to learn about the sadly neglected art of kissing.

I shall always remember my first sexy kiss, though I'm quite emphatic that at that time, I was fairly naive about sex. That first caress happened when lips sort of snuck up on me at a school dance. I must confess that the name of the schoolboy who administered it escapes me! At every organised school disco, the highlight of the evening came at that time late in the evening (probably around half past nine!), when the mood softened and smoochy records hit the turntable. Now this kind of smooching is in itself a very erotic act. The movement and positioning involved in close contact dancing can be an immense turn-on and even though I was not completely aware of the joys of sex, I knew that snuggling up cheek to cheek and groin to groin on the dancefloor felt very pleasurable indeed!

I remember my partner being an attractive teenager

I'd had my eyes on for some time. This naughty partner of mine was sliding a hard bulge that had developed in the front of his pants firmly into my crotch. His hands wandered up and down my spine before coming to rest on my arse. I thought it was immensely enjoyable, but a little embarrassing at first. I wasn't sure whether to slap him around the chops or reach down and give that inviting lump an encouraging little squeeze. Instead I stole a glance around the hall at my school chums, and noticed that they all seemed to be in exactly the same state. At that tender age, I didn't want to be thought too forward, so I merely thrust my hips back to meet his and waited for further developments.

They arrived in the form of my first real kiss. I think I was quite lucky in that respect, because I'm sure my schoolboy snogger had had previous experience. He placed one hand gingerly on my chin, tilted my face towards his, and softly put his lips to mine. It's amazing; I can't remember his name, yet I can recollect the warmth of his slightly moist, parted lips as they brushed against mine. There was no tongue-to-tongue contact at first, but nevertheless the sensation was extremely thrilling.

As one slow, sensual record slipped into another, our enthusiasm for canoodling increased. Ten minutes or so later, when we were still dancing with our bodies entwined, my partner let his tongue slip into my open mouth. Wriggling around exploratively, his tongue sought out mine, and I responded by plunging my tongue into his mouth. That's when the kiss really became spirited! All those sensitive little nerve endings rubbing against each other were bound to consume us both with passion. That was as far as it went, though; my dad picked me up after the dance and no heavy petting ensued!

46

From there I went from strength to strength, and now I can climax quite easily simply by kissing and rubbing myself against another similarly impassioned partner. The only penetration necessary is that of the tongue. It works best for me if I'm lying down, and on top of my lover – perhaps this is because in this position I can really get to grips with the necking; or possibly I get a kick out of being in control.

But that's enough about me. I talked to some mates about their kissing techniques and preferences. Georgette, a thirty-year-old marketing director, told me she wants more kissing!

Most of the men I meet seem more interested in fondling me, fingering me and fucking me than in kissing me, and I think it's a great shame. When I'm kissed, that's when it all starts happening for me. He holds me, he caresses my face and then he plants a kiss upon my lips. I love this and would prefer it if prior to lovemaking, men would spend more time simply embracing and kissing me. In my experience, most men will swiftly move on. I'm sure it's not because they don't enjoy kissing; possibly they believe you'll think them too slow if they don't reposition their lips on another part of your body pretty damn urgently. Don't get me wrong, I adore having every bit of my body kissed; I'd just like plenty of lip kissing prior to that!

Another thing that I have noticed about passionate kissing is that it's quite abundant in the early stages of a relationship, but frequently peters out. I can't understand why males seem to lose interest in erotic tongue kisses and move on to annoying little pecks instead.

My favourite way to begin making love is to be loosely clothed and to straddle my man on a sofa or large, comfy chair. I wrap my legs around his waist so I can feel his cock nudging between my open legs; then I take his face in my hands and initiate frantic, fiery kisses. I've usually climaxed long before we remove any clothing. Although I've been giving men a bit of a hard time and accusing them of not kissing girls enough, there are some brilliant, attentive kissers around. You just have to seek them out!

Wise words, Georgette; I agree wholeheartedly. We must not forget that sensual kissing is an erotic experience in itself and should never be neglected. As I've said many times before in this pleasure guide, if you aren't getting enough of whatever you fancy, tell your partner and talk it through. It may be only a misunderstanding or there may actually be a problem.

Of course if you want your lover to enjoy devouring and nibbling your delicate mouth, you must make sure that it's going to taste sweet. Visit the dentist regularly so that you don't contract any form of mouth or gum disease that causes bad breath. And of course clean and floss your teeth after meals. If you're a smoker and your lover isn't, I'd be tempted to say give it up, it's a disgusting habit. But I'd probably get severely criticised for that, so just be aware of how unpleasant the lingering smell of tobacco can be. Suck mints, chew gum or try to have a toothbrush or mouthwash on hand to dispel the acrid odour.

Now back to the snogging! Through persistent personal testing, I managed to seek out one of those extraordinary males who adores kissing. Gary hails from Essex, is thirty-five years old and divorced. He talks about the new love in his live: 'I adore kissing and cuddling. My girlfriend Sandra is an amazing kisser. Sometimes when we're kissing, I feel like I'm on cloud nine, savouring her sweet lips, exploring every inch of her mouth. Sometimes after a particularly good snog, we get sore lips because we're at each other's mouth for so long! When we fuck we almost always adopt positions in which we are facing each other so we can continue to kiss. I like to fuck her doggy-fashion, but we make love this way only occasionally because I really do miss that contact with her lips whilst we are fucking. When I am between her legs I use my tongue on her cunt to make her come, and as soon as she starts to climax she drags me up to her and crushes her lips to mine, so that we are kissing when she has her orgasm.'

I too enjoy that moment of exquisite pleasure, a simultaneous kiss and an orgasm. The other advantage of kissing a man after he's been licking your pussy is the lovely way he smells after he's been dipping his tongue into your honeypot. Another kind of kiss that hasn't yet been mentioned in this chapter are those sweet, tender kisses after either one or both of your have achieved your sexual zenith — those feverish bite-type kisses that you plant all over each other's mouth and face when you feel sated and exhilarated.

Hungry, exploratory kisses are also very important when building up to lovemaking. Your lover's lips are by no means the only area to concentrate upon. We girls like our men — or our lady friends for that matter — to kiss us on the neck or nibble on our ear lobes, although I could never see any great pleasure from receiving a wet tongue directly in my ear! But each to their own. It's a pleasure to feel a wet tongue slither across our throats and to savour those tiny planted love-kisses on our closed eyelids, nose and cheeks. Tease her with your lips until she's begging to taste your mouth. And of course, girls, the same applies to you. Men like to be made a fuss of, too.

As you know, I'm a keen advocate of erotica, or pornography as it is often labelled, but I do have some criticisms. In what is termed hard-core pornography we are rarely treated to a display of prolonged kissing. So come on, you porn producers, I for one would like to see plenty more tongue-to-tongue contact between that sexy male lead and his starlet. It seems to crop up much more frequently in lesbian and bisexual scenes but, dare I say it, I think that's because the majority of these films are made by men, for men, and men like to see girls kissing. What a pity they don't seem to derive as much satisfaction from watching a man and a woman! Naturally erotic movies feature plenty of body kissing, and I'd like to move on to explore other parts of the body and discover new erogenous areas.

Kissing the entire body is a quintessential part of lovemaking. It can almost take on the form of sexual worship. It should be done carefully and in a leisurely way, the lover taking his or her time to explore with the tongue and mouth. Work down from the mouth and let your tongue linger on the nipples. Spend time circling each one with gentle steady movements. Draw the nipple into your mouth and feel it swell. Naturally, while you are busy on the nipples your hands can be exploring other areas. Ladies, let your fingers dance across his scrotum, and guys, spread her legs and feel the furrow of her lips, dipping in between them to find her bud of flesh. Trace a delicate line of kisses to the bellybutton and move steadily over the belly. Then, very slowly, restraining yourself, descend towards the pubis. The idea is to prolong the sexual euphoria, so before going for gold explore the inner thighs, move along the perineum and seek out the anus. All these areas are extremely sensitive and will send you and your partner into tremors of passion, for it is not just the kissee that receives the ecstatic pleasures; the partner administering loving caresses with the tongue is duly rewarded by savouring the taste and the smell of their lover. And if they kiss with their eyes open there is even more to relish. As the lips move and the nostrils quiver, enjoy the fascinating spectacle that is your lover's body. Using your eyes is particularly arousing when it comes to oral–genital sex which we will explore explicitly in Chapter Five.

Aside from genitals and breasts, the inner thighs, the entire anal area, the armpits and the back are very special areas for most of us. Hand kissing can also be very suggestive. A moist tongue gently working on the palm of the hand or, as I've mentioned before, feasting on a finger, can certainly heighten sexual awareness. We mustn't forget our feet, either. Sucking on your lover's toes or running a gentle tongue between them can send them off into heady delirium. Actually it just makes me giggle, but that doesn't mean I don't enjoy it. Believe me, there's nothing wrong with having a good laugh when you're making love.

The key to successful body kissing is for both men and women to be gentle, careful and to take their time, with long, smooth, tender brushes of lips over flesh, suitably lubricated with saliva. The tempo can be varied and you should take your cue from your lover. Often women complain that men are too rough, so begin by sucking and licking her softly, building up to tiny bites and plucking a fold of flesh between your lips and drawing it into your mouth. She may love it or it might hurt. I know you've got your mouth full, but with body language you can work out what you both want!

Before starting on the next chapter, why not go away and practise the art of kissing? Then, when you've enjoyed a really good snog, strip your partner naked and work that tongue over their body. Pretty soon I suspect you'll be in the mood to sample a little fingering, squeezing and sucking.

LET'S RECAP!

- 'A sexual kiss is for me the commencement of foreplay. The first pleasurable moment when the union of lips begins the arousal process.'
- 'Most of the men I meet seem more interested in fondling me, fingering me and fucking me than kissing me!'
- 'When I am between her legs using my tongue on her cunt to make her come, as soon as she starts to climax, she drags me up to her and crushes her lips to mine.'
- 'The other advantage of kissing a man after he's been licking your pussy is the lovely way he smells after he's been dipping his tongue into your honeypot.'
- 'Guys, spread her legs and feel the furrow of her lips, dipping in between them to find her bud of flesh.'
- 'Sucking on your lover's toes or running a gentle tongue between the toes can send them off into heady delirium.'

4

Foreplay

A constant complaint from all kinds of women that I talk to is that an alarming amount of men are in a mad rush to perform — the old 'Wham, Bam, Thank You Ma'am' syndrome. I must admit there are occasions when foreplay doesn't interest me, those times when I urgently, almost desperately, want to be fucked — no kissing, no loving, no fingering, no sucking; all I yearn for is a good stiff cock probing between the folds of my cunt and ramming for home. But for most of the time this kind of animal behaviour leaves me high and dry. You know what I mean — when a man just wants a quick jump, wants to spread your legs and shove it right in there, with a quick tweak on your nipples as he pumps away mechanically. Perhaps they do it to impress? To show us just how much they want us? Perhaps I'm being too generous here. Maybe they're just downright lazy.

Thankfully these type of men are a small minority, and if I get hold of any of them I'll soon put them right. My advice would be — don't moan about it girls, change his ways or change your man! We should not have to put up with a man who shows no concern for our needs. In this age of equality, we may be as good as the fellas but we sure aren't similar in our make-up. Because a woman's body is completely different to a man's, we can enjoy numerous forms of sexual stimulation and often achieve multiple orgasms – in fact we can keep on coming until exhaustion or an inflamed genital region forces us to desist. When there are so many caring, sensitive, experienced males out there just waiting to be plucked, why should we put up with one quick lousy fuck?

It is imperative that as lovers we appreciate the importance of foreplay. The short-lived *Sunday Correspondent* newspaper did a survey which explored what women would want and expect from sex if they were to pay for it. I recall one woman's requirement was six hours of foreplay and a couple of hours of sexual intercourse, and I remember thinking I wish I'd said that!

In the last chapter we have explored the art of kissing and body kissing which can play a tremendous role in foreplay. Actually I don't know who the hell called it foreplay, but to me that suggests an activity that you just do before the big event, not before, during, and after. The kind of erotic play we term as foreplay continues throughout the lovemaking process. While my man is fucking me, it doesn't mean to say he's going to stop stroking my clit, squeezing my nipples and kissing my lips! I have one general rule that I usually impose on my male lovers; they have to make me come at least once with their tongue and fingers before I allow them to fuck me. I haven't had many complaints, and I do so love to hear a man beg!

It has to be said that during the sexual coupling, be it foreplay, fucking or what, the onus is on the man to perform and to satisfy his partner fully before he reaches his own peak. The apologies that I've had bestowed upon me by embarrassed men who have managed to give me only two orgasms to their one! Personally I prefer a ratio of three to one, but that's no big deal; with a little bit of foreplay, the cycle can start all over again, and again! We women are so lucky; your man may be completely shagged out, but if his fingers and tongue still have a bit of energy, we can drift off into pleasureland once more.

Let's get back to basics: the big build-up, the removal of clothes, the tender yet urgent kisses and caresses. During the early stages of your loveplay you can arouse each other without actually making contact with her bare pussy or his swelling prick. The term is frotting, and although I can't locate it in my dictionary it means the stimulation of touch through clothing. I'm not referring to getting touched up on the Northern line in rush hour by some frustrated weasel — no, I'm talking about the fondling of breasts through a tight sweater or lace bra, or the touch of fumbling fingers on a damp pussy through sheer silky panties. This is the way many girls experience their first orgasm with a partner; I know it was how I did. It was in the back of a Vauxhall Cresta with a boy who had his hands all over me, stroking my nipples through my bra and rubbing his quivering fingers up and down my slit through wet cotton panties. I wouldn't let him venture inside, but oh, did it feel good that very first time!

Frotting is a wonderful turn-on and a thrilling way to extend your loveplay. Here's an interesting letter that I received from Jess, who's found a new sexual lease of life as a frotteur!

I've recently remarried, and although my new wife Josie is a few years younger than me, she has really taught me how to make sex exciting. We were dating for a couple of weeks before I finally got to fuck her. In fact, up until that point in our relationship, we'd only indulged in goodnight kisses at the end of each date.

55

This particular night, we'd gone out to a restaurant and in the taxi on the way home she squeezed my cock through my trousers and whispered that she wanted me to take her home and make love to her. My response was: 'Yes please!'

We got to my flat, and as soon as we were in the doorway we started kissing passionately. She pulled away and asked me to sit down and watch her strip. My ex-wife had never gone in for any strip shows or sexy underwear, so you can imagine my delight when Josie whipped off her dress to reveal a matching set of flame-red undies complete with sheer black stockings. Her dark bush of black pubic hair was crammed into tiny lacy panties and her large nipples were hard and straining against the confines of her bra. As she stood facing me she snaked her hands all over her delicious body. I was so stunned I just couldn't say anything, but it had a dynamic effect on my body – my cock started to throb and swell.

On hands and knees Josie crawled over to me and began to stroke my bulge. She has beautifully manicured long fingernails and I shall never forget the feel of those red talons running gently along the length of my zipper, teasing my trapped cock. She suspended the excitement when she very steadily unzipped me. Now there was only one lot of material between her fingers and my swollen cock, as she played with me through my Y-fronts. I felt fit to burst, but I managed to control myself as she sensually squeezed my balls and let her fingers slip round towards my arsehole to play around there for a while. All the time I was fondling her breasts through her bra.

After a few moments of fiery passion, she

helped me off with my clothes and then, still dressed in her undies, straddled me on the couch. She grasped my cock expertly and stroked it along the tiny gusset of her knickers, which by now was soaking with her juices. The feel of the wet silk against the sensitive glans of my cock was incredible.

As Josie massaged my cock against her clit, I started to suck on her nipples through the bra. The lace seemed to give extra friction and I almost thought her nipples were about to break through the lace! She wanked the purple head of my cock against her cunt, which was still covered with that tiny strip of lace, until suddenly her body started to convulse. I held her tight as she cried out at the top of her voice. Her climax almost brought about mine, so I was relieved when she calmed down slightly, then swiftly pulled her knickers off to one side and sat down slowly on my cock. As she bounced up and down on top of me, I could still feel the damp lace rubbing against the base of my cock. She began to ride me, slowly at first, then faster and faster. With the teasing she'd given me I couldn't hold out for long, but that was fine, because as I felt my orgasm building, her pussy began to tighten around my shaft and she was coming all over again. Her contracting pussy walls finished me off and seconds later I was spurting and enjoying one of the most intense orgasms of my life. Now I spend a fortune on exciting undies for Josie to wear when we fuck!

It sounds to me as if Jess and Josie have a wonderful time in their loveplay. That very first session together was obviously a hot, hot night, but of course we shouldn't just let this exquisite, yet agonising build-up of sexual pleasure happen only in our first few sexual encounters with a partner. We can make each and every act of love a ceremony; whether our foreplay includes arousal by the use of explicit language, striptease, frotting, body kissing or mouthwatering oral sex, it should all add up to a hell of a good time. I've talked to lots of ladies about this and the conclusion I've drawn is that we girls want our lovemaking sessions to last even longer and for our men to be gentle. Not all females relish the idea of being fist-fucked or having their delicate little pussies used as a yardstick for a 'how many fingers can I stick in' competition! And make sure your fingernails are filed and clean — I love being fingered, but there's nothing more off-putting or uncomfortable than a man with dirty, scaggy nails.

Women like to be treated romantically, but that doesn't mean we want sex to be clinical and flowery! No, I like my moments of true passion to last for hours, sometimes to be unhurried, sensual and very dreamy; but other times I like them to be frenzied and downright dirty!

As lovers, we all have moods and through foreplay we should be able to gauge our parnter's sexual frame of mind. Now the way I rabbit on about sex, you might get the impression that I'm obsessed, and that I'm the kind of girl who craves it all the time, but there are occasions when I'm really not in the mood. But I've learnt that the times when I get turned on to it by a little gentle persuasion in the form of foreplay are often the best.

I recall one specific incident, when I'd had a trying day and I was feeling rather grumpy. My lover gave me a cuddle and very sweetly asked if he could have one quick glimpse of my puss just to keep him happy. I grudgingly agreed. He lifted my tight black dress (I was wearing no knickers at the time) and gasped at the sight of my golden love box. Then he asked me if he could possibly just touch my pussy for a second. So once again I frostily complied. I was laid on the bed with my dress pulled up around my thighs, my legs pressed tightly together as he very slowly rubbed one finger the length of my slit.

By now I was feeling very horny, but I didn't let on at all. In a very husky voice he begged that I let him taste me. I nodded my head curtly, managing to conceal my enthusiasm. His lovely hot tongue travelling up and down my parted pussy lips sent tingles up my spine, but still I kept my thighs firmly closed, making it more difficult for him, but even more exciting for me. In fact now it's a game I play with that particular fella quite often, not because I'm usually a sullen, grouchy ol' bugger, but just because I recall how good it felt as he tried to pry my legs open! It's wonderful the different games we can play to arouse our partners. I asked three different women to tell me what kind of foreplay turns them on.

Vicki, a model from London, told me: 'I like a man to be very tactile. I like holding hands, I love it if my man tickles my palm with his forefinger or, when he's holding my hand, starts to kiss it and then suck on one of my fingers. I adore intimate little glances and lingering caresses.

'When he takes me home I like to be stripped, very slowly and seductively. Being a model, I have some fabulous underwear and I love the feel of a man's warm hands removing it from my body, firstly easing my breasts out of my bra, slipping it from my shoulders as he kisses my neck and cups my tits. I've got very sensitive breasts and I love having my nipples sucked and squeezed quite hard. I like him to use his teeth to gently bite my nipples while his fingers explore the rest of my body; stroking my bottom, slipping his fingers

59

into the back of my knickers, running his fingertips along the furrow of my arse, down towards my cunt and making the first contact with it from behind. I love to hear a man's satisfied grunt when he first feels my cunt. They are always delighted to discover that I'm wet, because by this time I'm usually soaking. I like him to gently open my cunt and just tease me a little with his fingers, never quite going for my clitoris. Now I ask him to take off my knickers. I adore it when a man goes down on his knees and ever so slowly drags my panties from my hips halfway down my thighs. And, when my legs are trapped together within the restraints of the elastic, I long for him to smother my pubic hair with tongue kisses as I plead with him to eat me out.'

Sharon, another model from London, likes to use a mirror when she is getting ready for love.

'I'm proud of my body. I'm five foot nine inches tall, have a large bust, small waist and long legs. When I fuck with my boyfriend we both like to watch in the mirror. I love to get a close look as his meaty cock sinks into my twitchy twat. When we're ready for a fuck we like to take ages about it. Our favourite game of the moment is for me to lie on the floor in front of my full-length mirrored wardrobes, and play with myself while he watches. Sometimes I just use my fingers, plunge in as many as I can, or I use a vibrator, a hairbrush or whatever's handy. While I masturbate, he kneels beside me, sometimes kissing my mouth, playing with my tits until we both become so excited that we pounce on each other!'

A model from the North, called Lisa, revealed to me her favourite form of foreplay: 'The biggest turn-on for me is to actually start the foreplay while my boyfriend and I are out together, so that we have to wait until we're somewhere private to finish what we've started. For instance, I like to go to a restaurant and be played with under the table, or to take my bloke shopping and invite him into one of the individual changing rooms that you get in ladies' shops, on the false pretence of approving my clothes, when really all I want is for him to finger me! Even though we both have our own place, the amount of times we've fucked in the car because we've been unable to wait until we've got home is staggering.'

All three model girls sound like they're having fun to me! Perhaps you need a few tips or pointers to improve and prolong your loveplay, so I've listed half a dozen foreplay frolics for you to experiment with.

- Become a frotteur. Put on your best undies and let your partner play around with you through them. It feels damn good wanking a nice, stiff cock through a pair of silk boxers, and fingering a juicy fanny through moist material is an experience not to be missed.
- Take an agonising amount of time stripping each other of your clothing. Spend time caressing and stroking areas of the body that are often ignored; the shoulders, the neck, the back, the legs, the arms, the feet. Avoid any contact with the breasts and genital area until you are both frenzied with desire.
- When you are both stripped or semi-stripped, get to know each other's body intimately by kissing each other all over. Discover all the erogenous zones other than the genitals and really go to town with your lips, tongue and teeth.
- Girls, go out on the town with your man and forget your knickers. Don't let on till you're halfway through the evening, then whisper naughtily in his ear.
- Take a leaf out of my book, girls, and play it cool.

Tell him lazily when he starts getting fruity that you're not in the mood, but if he wants to try to turn you on, that's up to him! The knack is in the way you say it. If you really sound too disinterested he might just nip down the pub, so my advice is to throw a few smutty expletives in and tell him: 'Well, I'm not sure I want you to lick my pussy darling!' as you wriggle your arse around somewhat exotically and hoist your skirt up a modicum. Get my drift? This little ploy will also work for guys. She'll probably reward you with one of the most sensational blow jobs of your life, just to get you in the mood for love!

- Invent an erotic scenario, or borrow one from a book or magazine if necessary. Tell your lover in explicit detail how you've been dreaming of being fucked by the English rugby team or the Dagenham girl pipers — mock jealousy can be an unbelievable stimulant!

I think it's about time we moved along and savoured the delights of oral—genital sex — that, too, is an important part of foreplay. But before I draw this chapter to a close I'd just like to bring to mind some of those onomatopoeiac words that remind us of the joys of the flesh prior to full sexual coupling. Why not utter them out loud in a husky or breathy whisper to get you in the mood? Do make sure you're not standing at a bus stop at the time! Fingering, squeezing, sucking, tongueing, lapping, gorging, feasting, dribbling, squelching, gobbling, guzzling, oozing, salivating and slobbering. Now if that lot doesn't get your groin a-twitching, perhaps you'd better try the *Reader's Digest*!

LET'S RECAP!

- 'Those times when I urgently, almost desperately want to be fucked — no kissing, no loving, no fingering, no sucking. All I yearn for is a good stiff cock probing between the folds of my cunt and ramming for home.'
- 'We women are so lucky; your man may be completely shagged out, but if his fingers and tongue still have a bit of energy, we can drift off into pleasureland once more.'
- 'She grasped my cock expertly and stroked it along the tiny gusset of her knickers, which by now were soaking with her juices. The feel of the wet silk against the sensitive glans of my cock was incredible.'
- 'I love to hear a man's satisfied grunt when he first feels my cunt.'
- 'And when my legs are trapped together within the restraints of the elastic, I long for him to smother my pubic hair with tongue kisses as I plead with him to eat me out.'
- 'I love to get a close look as his meaty cock sinks into my twitchy twat!'

5

Oral Sex

'Head! That's what most of them ask for. I mean I don't see why a woman would have a problem sticking her man's cock in her mouth. I mean I guarantee you if he ain't sticking it in her mouth, he'll be sticking it in somebody else's.'

That's an interesting theory spouted from the sexy mouth of Theresa Russell whilst playing the leading role in Ken Russell's movie *Whore*. These wise words were taken from a stageplay written by David Hines, who gleaned all his information from actual prostitutes while transporting them in the back of his London taxi cab. If his observations are valid, which unfortunately I think they probably are, it's a sad indictment on today's supposed sexually liberated society if some women are still reluctant to perform the act of fellatio for their man, forcing frustrated males to turn to prostitutes as a substitute. And the boot can also be on the other foot. But sadly for us women, surrogate gigolos like dreamy Richard Gere are pretty thin on the ground! We women love the feel of a butterfly tongue tickling and teasing our chief pleasure zone but, believe it or not, there are some men out there who will not oblige. Not the kind of man I'll have anything to do with, mind you!

Satisfying and fulfilling lovemaking without

cunnilingus or fellatio would be difficult for me, as I have a particular penchant for both. Obviously there are times when the allotted time for love permits only a few stumbling fingers for lubrication purposes before it's straight down to business. And of course at times like those we don't participate in every act of love we desire, but as this pleasure guide is all about making the time and effort to enjoy sex to the full, then relaxing and enjoying both is a must.

Let's get to grips with fellatio first. Stimulating your lover's penis with your mouth is a very important and integral part of loveplay. And if you want to drive your man crazy in bed, then it's something you are going to have to learn about, girls. Practice makes perfect, and practising can be great fun! The very first time we slip that silky smooth member between our parted wet lips can cause slight embarrassment, not because there is anything unpleasant or offensive about letting his dick tickle your tonsils, but because women are afraid that they might not do it right! But persevere, girls, it's well worth it.

I recall with affection the first cock that I allowed to penetrate my sugar-sweet lips. It was backstage at a gig at the Johnson's Hall in Yeovil, Somerset with a rather well-hung bass player from a seventies rock band. He unzipped his outrageous yellow leather pants, flipped out this enormous fat cock and gave me a knowing look. I remember thinking, no way is that going to fit into my mouth! But it squeezed in nicely and in a smouldering, gravelly voice, he coaxed me through it, told me when and how to suck and the most sensitive areas to concentrate my tongue on, and he was then considerate enough to advise me in a very euphoric tone that he was about to splatter his lot all over my face! It was rather a pleasing initiation amongst the PA systems, musical instruments and rock paraphernalia. The most important lesson I learnt from that enlightening experience was always to gauge my partner's reaction, and how to savour the visual experience of studying the expression on my lover's face when I am turning him on, bringing him to boiling point and driving him crazy with my mouth.

So let's get down to tactics. When you first encounter his erect cock, hold it firmly at the base of the shaft and slide your tongue gently up and down its length. Take your time, and use your fingers to enhance the sensation. Don't fall into the trap of thinking that because you're sucking cock, you literally have to suck so hard you'd shift the chrome off a '56 Chevy! This sex act often gets called a blow job, but we seldom blow on it. Let your mouth fill with saliva and smother his cock with your wetness. Draw the glans in and out of your mouth and use your tongue to probe the tiny hole in the plumlike head. Pay attention to his balls, but be careful! Licking and sucking his scrotum must be a very delicate operation. Commence gingerly with long smooth movements with the tongue; never use your teeth unless he specially requests it and, unless you have a gigantic mouth, never attempt to cram both of his balls in at once. One at a time is the way I would recommend you proceed!

I mentioned to a couple of girlfriends that I was about to embark on a chapter concerning fellatio, and was offered these choice comments and reminiscences for inclusion.

Tricia, a mum of three from Wales, told me: 'My husband John is circumcised. He has a really beautiful prick and I love to suck on it. I still remember when we first met at a club and he offered me a ride home. I really wanted to fuck him, so as soon as we were in the car, I reached over and took his prick out. I thought it was so beautiful that I sucked him off right then and there. I asked him to switch the interior light on so that I could see what I was doing, make sure I was doing what he liked. I'd sucked a few pricks before tackling John's, so I had a good idea what I was supposed to do. Actually he told me afterwards that the fact that I made the first move and pulled his prick out of his pants so quickly turned him on more than ever. I think he also liked what I did to his prick, slipping my tongue up and down it, strumming his shaft with a fast flickering tongue while I gently squeezed his knob end with my fingertips. All the while he was holding my long black hair out of the way so that he could watch me sucking him off. In about two minutes flat he had spunked all over my face. That was the first time I'd ever let a man come in my face and the taste of his sperm came as a pleasant surprise.

'We've been married for over ten years now and we're still having a good time, and when I want to fuck, I know the way to get him going is to get out his prick and start sucking on it. It never fails!'

Lesley, a striptease artiste in her early twenties, told me how she injoys cocksucking: 'My boyfriend Gary is twenty-six years old and your regular type of guy. He likes me to dress up in stockings and suspenders, likes me to talk dirty to him when we fuck, and naturally likes me to suck his cock. That's fine by me, because I get turned on by all those things too. A special evening of sex usually starts with me going to work on Gary's cock. It works best for us if he's stripped naked and propped up on pillows on our large bed, and I kneel between his open legs. I find it a great turn-on to feel his cock grow in my mouth. I like to slip it in there when it's still quite flaccid and then just draw it in my mouth and feel it swell. With me, wanking and sucking go hand in hand, and sometimes I use baby lotion or oil which feels really good when rubbed on his hot throbbing cock. I've got used to the taste, so that doesn't bother me at all. I use my hands to slither up and down his rigid shaft, while I wriggle my tongue in his arse, lick all around his balls and then when he's begging for it, I go to work on his helmet again.'

Now I reckon both ladies have got the sucking situation well sussed. One female who hasn't sent me a letter regarding her hang-up. Suzanne wrote:

'I've been with my boyfriend for six months now and we've run into problems. I think I'm quite open about most things, including our love life. I thought we were having a pretty good time, but the other night it all came out. You see, Roger is disappointed that I don't enjoy taking him in my mouth. I just don't see what I'm supposed to get out of it. I've done it a few times, but I never seem to do it for long enough. There's no way I want to carry on until he comes in my mouth. If I did, where's the pleasure for me? I'd only have to suck him again to make him hard, so he would be able to make love to me. He also wants to lick between my legs and I'm not too happy about that. I suppose that I'd enjoy it if I let myself go, but I seem to have difficulty doing that!'

Lovemaking is all about give and take. Not just he gives you his dick and you suck it — it's far more complicated that that. Roger longs to feel Suzanne sucking him off, and why not? The poor guy is only human! She is perhaps too shy or just not willing to indulge him in his sexual desires, and I fear they may have come to a stalemate situation. No woman or man should ever be forced into doing something they are really not happy with whilst making love, but I would suggest that Suzanne try to loosen up or, as the hooker at the top of this chapter so rightly implied, Roger will be tripping off elsewhere to get his dick sucked.

I wrote back to Suzanne advising her to try to relax when she is having sex and not to take it quite so seriously. I assured her that there is a great deal of pleasure to be had from learning and loving the art of fellatio and that she should give it and her relationship a chance. And as she had admitted in her letter that she has on occasions awarded her lover's length the odd few licks, I suggested she get herself in a comfortable state of mind and give it a few more! I promised her it wouldn't bite! Then, once she's mastered that wondrous aspect of sex, she can lie back spellbound and be transported to cloud nine when Roger is finally allowed to explore between his lady's tightly clenched thighs.

Another sex act we ladies often aren't happy with is spunk-swallowing. Many women find it distasteful to swallow their lover's semen. I have one girlfriend who is a very well-known glamour model and an absolute tigress in bed — the type who would go for a night out, fancy two men and, unable to make a decision, take them both home and fuck the arse off them. She also likes the taste of pussy and is well into bondage, but ask her to drink a little come and the answer is a definite no. She told me that she's tried it, but it just makes her sick!

Personally I'm not enamoured by the taste, but I know how much it means to a man. The idea of being permitted to fill my mouth with his bulging cock as the first of his juices start to flow, his cock becoming even harder and more tense until finally he shoots his seed straight down my throat gives me a thrill because I know how much he adores it. Surely the fact that they have such a good time at it makes us want to try it one time? And, if you really don't like the taste, girls, you can at the last minute withdraw your mouth and allow his sperm to splash upon your face or perhaps

69

your breasts. I think it looks incredibly horny to see a woman with come dribbling from her lips — it's another of my favourite scenes from porno movies. Sperm is quite harmless and contains nothing more than protein and simple sugars. It has a slightly astringent taste that doesn't really linger, especially if you wash it down with a good Chablis. Give it a go, girls. It makes him feel complete and just think what you can persuade him to do for you while he's feeling so hot!

I visited Los Angeles earlier this year to interview some of the top Hollywood porno stars. One question that I was intent on asking them was how the hell do they deep throat? I know exactly what it is in theory — a similar trick to sword-swallowing! The head must be held well back so that the mouth and throat are positioned more or less in a straight line. Try as I might to line up an engorged member deep into my throat, I always end up gagging. Apparently for a man it is a truly unbelievable sensation and if you can get it right, it's pretty amazing for females too, so I am still keen to master the art. Here's a few tips from the girls who know:

Porsche Lynn, a statuesque redhead with a body like a Las Vegas showgirl, told me her views on deep throating: 'It's all down to the size of the guy's cock. It not only has to be the right size, but the right shape as well. If it fits, I do it. When I suck cock, I use a lot of wetness, use both hands and give a lot of attention to the balls.'

Sharon Mitchell, star of over two thousand hard-core movies, said: 'Vanessa Del Rio taught me to deep throat with a banana. If you could get it down without breaking the banana you were doing real good. The position that works for me is lying on a bed with my head hanging off the edge, then the cock sinks slowly into my mouth and throat from above.'

Savannah, probably the hottest new starlet on the erotic film scene, talked a lot, but didn't really assist me in my quest: 'I just love big dicks, the bigger the better. Big dicks make me come. I do deep throat really well. I don't know how it works, but it just goes all the way down. It just slides on down my throat, I don't know how!'

As you can probably gather, after much probing I'm still not much the wiser. I have established that the shape and size of the dick is very important, so I will keep on looking for that elusive, perfectly shaped penis. I shall get comfy and lie down with my head flopping over the edge of my bed, once in possession of a large shipment of West Indian bananas, and if all else fails, keep on sucking on my forefinger until I get it right!

Soixante-neuf. Or sixty-nine, for those of you who refuse to adopt French phrases. It's funny, but I can never think of that number without sexual connotations leaping to mind — that joyous sex act of simultaneously pleasing each other orally. Again I'm going to offer my four penn'orth. I'm really not to keen on it. Give me an attractive stiffy to feast on and I'm happy for hours, and if I've a man with an enthusiastic tongue with a talent for using it let loose between my hot little thighs, he'll be lucky to get out within a fortnight. But doing both at the same time? It just doesn't work for me. It's rather like patting your head and rubbing your tummy. When I'm sucking on a cock, I really want to give it my all, use my mouth, my tongue, both hands, baby oil, the works. I love to watch my lover's face, I like to examine every inch of his cock and even watch myself in action in the mirror — you know, really give it my best shot and concentrate on the job in hand. And equally when I'm spreadeagled across my four-poster, my legs tethered to the bedposts, my labia

71

majora gaping, my clit engorged and swelling, I just want to be licked and lapped and loved, to close my eyes and let those multiple orgasms wash me afloat in my own ocean. Get my drift?

Now, put the two together and for me it just doesn't happen. But if you're one of these people who's good at concentrating your attention on two things at once, then climb aboard, and roll and romp from one position to another, and savour each other's delicacies. If sixty-nine is your favourite number, feel, taste and smell your way to your sexual zenith.

Moving on to a subject that is very dear to my heart, and for that matter to the hairy haven pulsating between my legs as well – pussy-eating, licking her out, Frenching, going down on, cunt-lapping, muff-diving, honeypotting, kissing the pink, and plating, to name just a few of the affectionate terms often used to describe cunnilingus, the art of making us girlies go weak at the knees and quiver with delight. So, if the lady in your life requests any of these aforementioned, you'll know exactly what she's after. Personally I love it; in fact, I'm such a keen advocate of cunnilingus that when asked about my ideal man, a long eager tongue is the first quality that springs to mind.

I think that the most important rule for men who want to be good at this rapturous sport is to be unhurried and gentle. If we want you to suck harder on our clit, lap faster at our juices or probe your tongue deeper into our hot little lovehole, we'll let you know. And girls, if he gets a bit too rough in his excitement, tell him, just as you must tell him when a particular caress with his tongue starts to build towards a climax. Describe to him just how good it feels. Tell him quite graphically. In my experience men are turned on by dirty talk, and I know it gets me carried away. And guys, when you go down on her, don't go for gold straight away. Make her wait. Tease her a little. Use lots of saliva and concentrate on that area just to the right or left of her pussy. Wriggle your tongue along the inside of each thigh. Then in one big sweeping motion of the tongue lick her from her anus to the top of her slit before homing in on her lovebutton. Use your hands to open her lips, or slide a finger inside. For a change of angle, insert your thumb instead of a finger. That way your fingers are nicely placed for further stimulation. Reach up and cup a breast, squeeze her nipple or grab handfuls of her flesh around the pubic hair region. Slide back up her body and kiss her hard on the lips. Let her enjoy the smell of her sex that lingers on your mouth.

Of course, cunnilingus plays a major role in bisexual and lesbian relationships, and I will be covering that area in some detail later. But here I thought it worth mentioning a few quotes from females who reckon that the fairer sex are often more proficient at oral loveplay because they realise what a delicate, sensitive area the vulva is.

Tina, a shop proprietor from Kent, said: 'Sometimes my boyfriend gets so carried away when he's going down on me that he actually hurts. I have to grab him by the ears and calm him down! With my girlfriend I never have that trouble.'

Sarah, an actress, told me: 'Having my pussy eaten is wonderful if the guy knows what he's doing. If he doesn't, then you could be in for a rough time! I'm bisexual and when I let my girlfriends eat me out, I find I often have to ask them to lick me harder and faster.'

When I asked one friend of mine what advice she would like to give to men to improve their technique for oral sex, her answer was short, concise and straight to the point: 'Tell them not to use their teeth!'

So in conclusion, fellas, treat her pussy like the little flower that it is. If she likes to play a little rough, I'm sure she'll demand that you treat her a little more aggressively! And remember, designer stubble might look pretty neat but it doesn't feel so hot!

While we are on the subject of shaving, why not ask her to shave off all her pubic hair? Bald is beautiful when it comes to cunts. I found it a completely new sensation when around five years ago I shaved my pussy for a modelling session. When the job was over I had a great deal of pleasure with my pussy stripped of its usual golden thatch. It just looked so rude. I was like a kid with a new toy! It had to go basically because the readers of *Club International* magazine desired me unveiled, and being an acquiescent kind of girl, I was only too happy to oblige. At the time I was working as a columnist for that particular men's mag, and was inundated with mail that pleaded and begged for me to have a close shave. So it had to go!

I remember returning home to my boyfriend after the photo session. I was wearing a shorty dress, stockings, suspenders and no knickers. When I walked in the door, he was all ready for me. He knew that I'd be hot to trot because I'd spent all afternoon exhibiting my bald beauty to the camera. I hitched up my dress and he went down on his knees to give my hairless hole a good tongue-bashing. And fucking was sensational too. I let it grow back, though, because shaving it every day was a real bore. Now I just trim the crown and depilate my lips. My pussy looks like something out of a Hollywood porno movie!

I recieved a letter from Ray in Scotland who wrote to me about his penchant for shaven havens.

'I would like to ask why genital depilation is the exception rather than the rule. Surely I cannot be the only man who finds a hairy vulva the biggest turn-off. Having recently met a woman who keeps herself completely free of pubic hair, my previously inhibited sex life has changed dramatically. Now I can and do spend hours licking her, which is a great source of pleasure for both of us. Why are women so reluctant to shave themselves and bare all?'

Why indeed? Perhaps it's because we girls don't want to get into the habit of shaving every day, but I suspect it's because many women feel uncomfortable without their thick bush of hair to hide behind. Persuade her to shave it off just the once, and while you're at it, why not get rid of yours as well?

The penis and vaginal area are not used solely for pleasure. They are of course a means of expelling urine from our bodies and in addition to this can be cooped up in tight clothing for the biggest part of the day, so hygiene is of the utmost importance. Who the hell will put up with licking and sucking a sex organ that doesn't smell too good? The penis is often accused of being cheesy and the vagina of being fishy. These pungent smells are not a subject I wish to dwell on!

Let's deal with the vagina first. Now the vagina has a very good cleaning system all of its own, but that doesn't mean you shouldn't wash it regularly. If you aren't fortunate enough to have a bidet, one way to douche yourself in an efficient and pleasing manner is to lie in the bath tub, spread your legs and aim the shower nozzle at your open lips. It is also necessary to wash the vulva thoroughly. The clitoral hood should be lifted to be cleansed. A quick splash of soap and water will not do. But be careful not to overdo it, girls! I think we women are often guilty of bathing and douching too much and then we wash away that beautiful heady smell that is our own natural aroma. I like to dab a little toilet water around the top of my inner thighs, but I advise that you keep the perfume light and away from your lips and clitoris. For one thing, a strong perfume removes your own essential odour, and also it burns like hell!

A circumcised penis is easiest to keep fresh, clean and a joy to be gobbled! I like them best anyway. Use lots of soap and water up and down the shaft, paying attention to the head, balls and anus. For fellas complete with a foreskin, just ease it back and wash thoroughly. I recommend washing twice a day for both sexes. I know this might sound like I'm a bit of an expert at stating the bleeding obvious, but you'd be amazed at some of the horror stories I've heard!

Now that you are both so clean and fresh and know the basics of oral–genital sex, I think you're just about ready to push on to the next enthralling step, that fabulous state of ebullience when penetration is inevitable, when animal lust has you firmly in its grasp, and you are indeed ready for love . . .

LET'S RECAP!

- 'I don't see why a woman would have a problem sticking her man's cock in her mouth. I mean I guarantee you if he ain't sticking it in her mouth, he'll be sticking it in somebody else's!'

- 'Sperm is quite harmless and contains nothing more than protein and simple sugars. It has a slightly astringent taste that doesn't really linger, especially if you wash it down with a good Chablis.'

- 'I'm such a keen advocate of cunnilingus that when asked about my ideal man, a long, eager tongue is the first quality that springs to mind.'

- 'If I've a man with an enthusiastic tongue and a talent for using it let loose between my hot little thighs, he'll be lucky to get out within a fortnight!'

- 'When I asked a friend of mine what advice she would give to men to improve their technique for oral sex, her answer was short, concise and straight to the point: "Tell them not to use their teeth!" '

- 'Bald is beautiful when it comes to cunts!'

6

Ready for Love

Now you are both so turned on, it's time to fuck!

I suppose we can all remember vividly the first time we had sexual intercourse and for the vast majority of us, if we're truly honest, the earth didn't move. Of course in the early stages of coupling we are nervous and somewhat embarrassed, and sometimes we females even feel a little pain. Losing one's cherry gets even more complicated if you're both novices. In my case the guy who took my virginity in the back of his band's transit van was twenty-seven and knew exactly what he was doing! I recall the kissing, cuddling and touching as very exciting, but the act of intercourse was a non-event and it hurt!

I asked a few people to tell me about the first time they had sex. One deflowered virgin, Sadie, a leggy blonde model from Texas, revealed: 'I was still at school and living in Texas. Two girlfriends and I went over to this boy's house, that one of my friends liked. So we went over there and this guy got us really drunk. Then he told me we should lay down for a while. I was happy to, the room was spinning. The next thing I knew he had us all in his bed with no clothes on. I can't even remember fucking! I was just a bit sore and terrified that my mother was going to find out. I went home with alcohol on my breath and no cherry!'

Gerry, a nineteen-year-old chef from Surrey, said: 'I was so worried about doing it for the first time. The pressure is really on. But I was going out with this girl who was slightly older than me, and I knew she expected it. We did it at her house and it was all quite romantic. We undressed each other and because I was so excited I had a steaming great erection. She lay down on the sofa with her legs spread and guided me into her. The first feel inside her cunt was electric. I had to start thinking of all kinds of things to stop myself from coming straight away. It didn't really work, though, and I came within two minutes!'

Brittany, a twenty-eight-year-old dancer from Detroit, told me her story: 'I was sixteen years old and it was my birthday. I was very sexually promiscuous in my early teens, I did just about everything but fuck – hand jobs, oral sex – but I was very aware of getting pregnant. There were a lot of pregnant teenagers in Detroit. But I decided on my sixteenth birthday that this was gonna be my time. It was after the high school football game with one of the players and it was in the front of a Cadillac Eldorado. We didn't make it to the back seat! It was pretty good. I didn't come, but it felt nice!'

Lesley, a kissogram girl from Essex, was a quick learner: 'I was very young and didn't have any experience at all, but I did know what it meant to be a virgin. My friends were always telling me to try it because I'd love it, so that really made me think about it. Every night I'd lie in my bed playing with myself thinking about it. So finally I was babysitting and this boy that I really liked came round. Before that night, we had kissed and I'd let him play with my tits, but that was all. That night when he started to stick his hand up my skirt, I let him. It felt good when he touched my fanny. We ended up screwing on the living-room floor. I remember it being really painful and it didn't happen for me at all. So the next day we tried it again and this time it did happen!'

Lesley seems to have got it right very quickly, as even experienced lovers take a little time to perfect the art of lovemaking. The fact that you are unfamiliar with each other's bodies can add to the excitement − that first thrilling touch and the tremble of anticipation are wonderful − but it does have its down side. After those tender kisses, fumbling fingers and plenty of oral to accustom yourself to your new partner, you must decide on a position that is arousing and with which you both feel comfortable. In addition, it is also important to adopt a position that helps the penis to stimulate the clitoris. The speed and rhythm of your lovemaking can vary considerably and there's nothing worse than a lover who is frantically pumping when he should be picking up his momentum slowly and leisurely. Discuss the speed and friction that is right for both of you. I like to start at a snail's pace and build to something that compares to a speeding express train!

When the act of penetration is about to take place, it's a nice gesture to assist entry of the erect cock into your eager pussy. Hold it just below the head, near the top of the shaft, and if he has a foreskin make sure that it is well peeled back. Perhaps use your other hand to spread your lips and welcome him inside. To prolong the pleasure, he may want to tease you a little by rubbing the swollen head of his engorged cock just inside the vulva without actually sliding it inside. This is a wonderful sensation and helps immensely with extra lubrication. You can never be too wet, I think.

As he plunges into you for the first time, thrust

your hips back to meet with his so that his cock goes deep inside you. His pubis bone will rub against your clitoris and you'll be able to feel the slap of his balls at the bottom of your slit. And guys, tease her even more; just when she's having a great time feeling you all the way inside her, slip it almost all the way out. Let her feel the head throbbing just inside the lips of her pussy, then, with a firm push, thrust it all the way in again.

Many women don't realise how much they can control their pleasure during intercourse. For instance, if you are in the missionary position and he is resting on his elbows thrusting inside your pussy, and you want to feel him deeper inside you, all you have to do is spread your legs a little wider and elevate them. His cock will now slide into you even further and at a more acute angle. If you wrap your legs around his back and thrust upwards to meet him, his cock should end up nudging your cervix, which will feel delightful for both of you. And don't forget that if you really want to squeeze his cock, clench your vaginal muscles when he's right up inside you. That will give him one hell of a thrill! If you're not quite sure how to control these important muscles, turn to the chapter on erotic exercises and you'll soon have the know-how.

Sexual intercourse can last all afternoon or all evening if you have the time. Most males are terribly considerate and prefer us females to have a jolly good time before they come. I was quite amazed when a boyfriend told me that he started thinking about boring book-keeping work to stop him from spurting too soon! If your lover does feel a frantic urge to come, you can help him, not by quoting your latest VAT output but simply by parting your legs so that there is less pressure on his penis, and by slowing up the movements of your hips. He should be able to slow down with you and prolong the pleasure.

Ideally, making love should be unhurried and relaxed. There should be no rules; just do what feels good for both of you. Luckily for women, most men are just as concerned for their partner's orgasm as they are their own. I think it's better if the female is manipulated or licked to her first orgasm prior to penetration; then, if he really can't stop himself from coming and she's not quite ready, well, she's happy anyway. And of course once he's come, it's only a matter of a little mouth-to-cock resuscitation to get his dick up again, because there really is nothing like a simultaneous orgasm!

If you start off in the missionary position and you fancy a change, roll over and let her ride on top. Allow his cock to slip out and bend over to savour the delights of rear-entry penetration as he fucks you doggy-fashion. That's why sex on a large king-size bed is such fun – there are no limitations on positioning. Enjoy making love in as many positions as you like, although one thing I would advise that, when you are almost there, just about to feel that white-hot flash streaking through your body and manifesting itself in one almighty orgasm, you need to be comfortable, to be able to close your eyes and let the spasm of ecstasy wash over you. You don't really want to be swinging from the chandeliers or sliding down the banisters!

Now there's been a lot written about the various ways of having sex, but in my book there are really only five standard positions.

MAN ON TOP OF WOMAN
This is probably our first introduction to sexual intercourse, and because it is not terribly adventurous

is often looked upon with scorn by the so-called advanced lovers. It is actually a very satisfactory position for lovemaking. The pelvic movements can be controlled and face-to-face kissing and caressing is possible. The penetration in this position is not especially deep unless the female elevates her bottom and wraps her legs around her man's back.

WOMAN ON TOP OF MAN

The Yanks call this the 'cowgirl' position and I guess you can see what they mean. The woman faces the man and rides him. She can also squat on her haunches with her back to him, or kneel over him and slide up and down him that way, or actually lie flat out on top and squeeze her legs together. Wriggling around on top you can come up with all kinds of stimulating variables. Some of you might find it a bit strange being there on top, taking charge as it were, but you'll soon get used to it, and being in this dominant role means you can dictate the pace and also achieve very deep penetration. And a pair of rounded tits bouncing up and down in front of your lover's face is a great pleasure for him.

LYING SIDE BY SIDE

Now this always reminds me of a lazy fuck. Not one that isn't enjoyable, but one that just happens when you're all cuddled up and something big and stiff starts poking you in the rear! For obvious reasons, this is often referred to as 'spooning'. You lie in front of your man and he tucks up behind you. This is an extremely comfortable position in which to make love, and your man can stroke your breasts and play with your clitoris from behind. The main disadvantage is that you can't really build up much of a forceful rhythm, because if he fucks you with much vigour you end up being pushed away from him.

WOMAN ON BACK, MAN ON SIDE

This is an interesting one because the male slides his member into the vagina sideways as he raises his partner's legs. This position is often called the scissors and the unusual angle of entry is very exciting for both lovers. In addition, the man has a free hand to caress the women's breasts and clitoris, and she can play with his balls or feel his cock as it slides in and out. The problem here is that the man can easily get exhausted!

WOMAN KNEELING, MAN ENTERING HER FROM BEHIND

We all know and love the doggy position. The female either kneels on all fours or kneels up, and the man enters her from behind. This is another deep-penetration position, and if she is on all fours, the man can feel the woman's breasts. This position is especially good for hard, energetic sex, and one added pleasure is the slap of the man's balls as he hammers his cock into his lover. But if the man has a large cock and the woman is small, this position can feel uncomfortable for her, especially if the man lifts himself by kneeling on one leg only, placing his raised leg flat-footed on the floor.

You can both use your imagination to come up with new ways to make love. Try standing up against the wall, or letting her sit down on your cock while you sit on a hard-backed chair. Any position, whether standing, sitting or lying, will involve some variation of these five basic positions.

I find it difficult to select my favourite sexual position, but I do enjoy the missionary position because it allows me play with my partner's cock and balls as he fucks me, and I can kiss him forcefully on the lips when I am coming. My personal preference is to vary the position by elevating my arse, raising my legs and wrapping them tightly around my partner's back, enabling him to fuck me really hard. One other position that always gives me great satisfaction is when I am on top, not sitting up or squatting on my haunches but lying flat out. In that position my clitoris receives maximum stimulation.

I asked several of my female friends and colleagues their preferred positions for making love. Here are some of the replies:

Louise told me: 'My favourite sexual position is spoons, I love the feel of it. You know when you lie on your side and he comes right behind you and slides it into you. It's the best because you can feel every inch of it. That position gets me off so easily.'

Claire couldn't decide. 'I have two favourites. I like doggy, because it's like *wham!* and I'm there. It's like slamming it hard into me, so I can't get away. I also love it if you get me on my back and put my knees right back by my ears. Now that's a good one!'

Tracy likes to be in control: 'I would say when I'm riding on top, sitting down on his cock, facing him. I like that because I can control how much and where I take it in my pussy. When I swing round from that position so my back is facing my bloke, it's pretty nice too.'

Rachel revealed: 'My favourite position is standing up against the wall. That's fun. I like it best with me leaning against the wall, with the man against me with his whole body. He has to be taller than me, though!'

Mandy said: 'I like to be on my back on the couch with my boyfriend in front of me and my legs over his shoulders. That's really my favourite one. That just hits the spot.'

I would say from experience that an average man comes twice when making love, and whereas some only need a matter of minutes to achieve an erection again, others need more time. (An old boyfriend told me how he once stayed inside a girl and managed to come three times, one straight after the other, without any stimulation other than his partner's hip movements. As he was only about twenty at the time and he's now in his late thirties, the details of how he managed it are foggy!) But I'm not saying that a man who ejaculates twice whilst making love is the norm, because as we know we are all different and some men are completely exhausted and fulfilled with one explosive orgasm. These particular males generally control their lovemaking and often withdraw their penis partway through sexual intercourse to concentrate on oral sex or manual stimulation. On the other hand, however, I've known men to come more than half a dozen times. Some can even match me climax for climax, and that takes some doing, me being a multiorgasmic kind of girl! You know the type of fellas I mean — the ones who make it difficult for us to get up and walk away afterwards without looking like we've a horse between our well-spread thighs!

While we're on the subject of bow-legged females, let's consider dick size. Now I think it's a fallacy that women have trouble shutting their legs after sampling a mammoth monster, and I also think it's pure fantasy that women long for a big dick. Men seem to be so self-conscious about their cocks, in the way some women are about the size of their breasts. We should all try to come to terms with the way we look. I don't really go along with the idea of having one's tits enlarged. Lots of my friends who are models have had it done and usually it looks great, but I'm sure they must lose some of their sensitivity and I wonder how their false breasts will look in the year 2000? In the States you can now have your dick pumped up as well! But let me put you straight on dick size, guys. What women really long for is a considerate lover who knows how to use his dick, his hands and his mouth. Now big dicks are fun, but so are medium-sized ones, and tiddlers can be good also, as long as the owner hasn't got a hang-up about having such a small dick!

I've been working on a movie set recently and in the breaks between filming I asked some of the girls on set how they like their cocks.

Julia, a stunning twenty-seven-year-old brunette model, said: 'Actually I prefer them small and I've married an animal. Is he human? Usually I prefer them smaller because I'm teeny-tiny inside.'

Chris, a make-up artist in her thirties, told me: 'Some of the best lovers I've ever had have had small cocks. Fucking isn't about just sliding a cock into a pussy. Sure, a big cock looks the nicest when you suck on it, but sometimes there are certain positions that I can't fuck in if the guy is hung like a donkey!'

Tina, a twenty-five-year-old hairdresser, admitted: 'I don't want to disappoint small men, but I like them big. It doesn't matter if they're thick or not, but I like them long, because I like to feel it in me really deep. Also when you're turning on to sex, the whole idea that you're going to get fucked by this great big cock — well, it's a turn-on in itself.'

In the next few chapters we shall be looking at ways to enhance your lovemaking further — ways such as dressing up for sex, acting out your fantasies, making love in all sorts of weird and wonderful locations and even the kinkier side of love. But now, before I go on to talk about possible problems and variations on genital sex, I would be a very naughty girl if I didn't expound upon the importance of safe sex. AIDS is a disease that we all know about only too well. But many men and women consider that unprotected heterosexual sex with a new partner isn't a risk. Well, it is, and the sooner we come to terms with that, the sooner we can attempt to arrest the problem. Having full sexual intercourse without a condom is not practising safe sex. Now if you've already found your perfect partner and are not busily auditioning for the leading role in your love life, well fine; but if not, be responsible and stock up on rubber johnnies. They come in all sorts of colours, thicknesses and flavours and they must be eased on to the male member before any penetrative sex takes place. You know it makes sense!

As with all fun activities that award us pleasure, things don't always go so smoothly. What if his dick goes soft whilst lovemaking? Or he ejaculates immediately or even before he enters you? Well, you can be your own sex therapist, you know. The first step is to sit down together and admit to each other that you've got a problem that you need to work at. There could be all sorts of reasons why his dick has gone limp during intercourse — too much alcohol, for instance, or perhaps tiredness. The way to deal with it is not to try to continue fucking. Let him withdraw and pay attention to his cock, either manually or orally. Try to wank or suck him to erection again. Once his cock is hard again, guide it back into your vagina and carry on where you left off. Whatever you do, don't get irritable or show disappointment, because that's one sure way to keep him floppy.

Premature ejaculation is something else that you can both work at to correct. Many men suffer from this because of early sexual experiences, trying to come quickly in case Mum comes home and catches you wanking or shagging the girl from next door on the sofa. It is also a problem for chauvinistic men, who have often been brought up to believe that sex is for men to enjoy while women lie back and think of England. The whole point of their sexual encounter is for them to reach orgasm, and as a result, they ejaculate quickly, leaving their partners high and dry. Obviously the female of the partnership is not happy, and the whole relationship can go down the drain. But if your lover ejaculates prematurely there is a good chance he can be cured. When taking on the role of sex therapist, patience and a caring attitude are imperative. Don't get angry or frustrated; just put aside some time together to talk and work the problem through.

The first step towards overcoming the problem of premature ejaculation is pleasuring. Strip naked and lie beside your partner on the bed. Return to the joys of foreplay and take your time kissing and caressing; no penetration or ejaculation must take place. Let him pleasure you while you relax and enjoy the sensations. Then return the compliment.

After several sessions like this you will both be ready to move on. The next step is to learn to grip your lover's penis in such a way that you control his urge to ejaculate. Place the round of your thumb under the opening in the head of his penis and then put two fingers around his shaft, one on top of the ridge around the head and one just below. If you squeeze him firmly in this way you will stop him coming and will not hurt him. Once you've learnt to control his climax by squeezing him when he's bubbling up to an orgasm, you are ready to fuck! Get him to lie flat on his back and lower yourself on to him. Don't jerk up and down; just keep very still. If he informs you that he is about to come, take it out and give it a squeeze before sitting down on his cock once again. Let him get used to having his cock inside you. Hopefully from that stage on you will be able to ride him slowly. I would suggest that when you are going to make love, get him to arouse you with his tongue and fingers until you are on the brink of coming, then when you do straddle him, if he comes quite quickly, you will be ready to orgasm as well.

Anal sex, fist-fucking and tit-fucking should all get a mention in this chapter. Having quite a firm pair of bosoms myself, I'm quite fond of tit-fucking. Here's a snippet from a letter I received from Nicole, a self-confessed nymphomaniac tit-fucker:

By the time we made it to Robert's bedroom it was still only early evening, so we had plenty of time to make this a night to remember. I instructed Robert to make himself comfortable on a chair a few feet from his bed while I went into my routine. Robert's eyes fixed on my body as I knelt on all fours on his bed, faced him and gave him an eyeful of my swinging tits still caged in my bra and dress. I moved from left to right to allow him to watch them sway from side to side.

'Want to see?' I teased.

Silently he moved his head up and down. His hands were already unzipping his flies.

I dropped both shoulder straps of my dress and, sitting back on my heels, I started to squeeze my tits through my bra. My erect, pink nipples peeked through the lace.

Robert now had his big, fat cock in his hand and he was stroking his shaft very slowly.

'Nice and easy!' I breathed as I undid the clasp on my bra. Proudly I took out my boobs one at a time. As I did I could hear Robert groaning. I pushed both of my heaving hooters together and massaged them vigorously. Then I bent forward on all fours so he could watch them hang down.

'Like to shove that big dick between these?' I offered.

Robert was on his feet. Together we discarded his trousers and pants and I lay back on the bed as he got to grips with my tits. First he used both hands to push them together, kneading them enthusiastically, his tongue frantically licking them, burying his face in my gigantic 38 DDs. I could feel his stiff cock probing my tummy to remind me of the delights to come as he feasted on me like a starving man.

'Let me feel those balls slapping against my tits!' I urged.

Robert was there in a second, holding my bouncing bazookas in position as he jerked his cock between them. His fat dick was already moist as it poked into the heavenly chasm fashioned from my wobbling tits. He thrust it back and forward, faster and faster, until I felt a hot gush of sperm slide between my sweaty slappers and come to rest on my neck. Robert released his dick in a frenzy and let the last few spurts ooze over my engorged pinky nipples.

After perusing that letter, I expect you'll agree that tit-fucking sounds like a lot of fun, and remember, it also conforms to the rules of safe sex. One sexual activity that doesn't is arse-fucking. It should never really be attempted by anyone who cannot open their arse easily to take insertion; otherwise too much stress is put on the condom and it will probably split. Of course if you're in a long-term relationship with no fear of AIDS, fucking up the arse is an alternative way to have sex. Pressure should never be put on a woman to indulge in this practice − a little gentle persuasion and lots of KY jelly is better! The whole process should be slow and gentle. The woman must relax to dilate her arse and the man must probe inside her inch by inch. When enjoying anal intercourse you might like to slide a vibrator into the pussy. There is only a thin wall separating the rectum and vagina, so the buzzing of the sex aid can give you both an added thrill. Many women are quite proud to use both their anus and vagina for lovemaking, and guys seem to get a tremendous kick out of this taboo practice.

Finally we turn to fist-fucking. This sexual act has become very big on the gay scene. The idea is to clench your fist and insert it as far as possible into either the vagina or the rectum. It sounds pretty barbaric to me, and can be harmful to your intestines. With regard to safe sex it's risky if you have any nicks or cuts on your hands. Try three or four fingers and give her a good tonguing instead − it sounds far less dangerous and much more fun to me! And after all, having fun with sex is what this pleasure guide is all about.

LET'S RECAP!

- 'The first feel inside her cunt was electric. I had to start thinking of all kinds of things to stop me coming straight away.'
- 'To prolong the pleasure, he may want to tease you a little by rubbing the head of his engorged cock just inside the vulva without actually sliding it inside.'
- 'I was quite amazed when a boyfriend told me that he started thinking about boring book-keeping to stop him from spurting too soon!'
- 'Once he's come, it's only a matter of a little mouth-to-cock resuscitation to get his dick up again.'
- 'I've known men to come more than half a dozen times. Some can even match me climax for climax which takes some doing, being a multiorgasmic kind of girl!'
- 'His fat dick was already moist as it poked into the heavenly chasm fashioned from my wobbling tits.'

7

Dressing Up for Sex

There's something deliciously decadent about being screwed over the living-room table with a posh evening frock wriggled up over your arse, your damp, lacy black knickers wrenched off to one side, one of your stocking-clad legs raised up, your high-heeled patent court shoe digging into the hard-backed chair as he slaps his cock ferociously between your vibrating arse cheeks, his smart trousers dropped around his ankles. Now this particular sexy scenario usually happens when you've been out on the town with the man in your life and you're all dressed up to the nines, you've both had a few to drink, and the pair of you are feeling horny. Or you're out on the razzle and you've pulled.

'Wait till I get you home!' he'll promise as you slip away early and hurry homeward bound. Withing a few seconds of being in your abode, it's trousers down, tackle out, let's fill up that damp pussy with something good, solid and meaty!

But on the evenings we don't venture outside our cosy little home, do we slop around in a grubby dressing gown and slippers? Yes, I think we often do, and that probably isn't going to have the desired effect. Well, OK, we all want to be comfortable, so I'm not advocating that you sit down and watch *Coronation Street* in your Sunday best. But do remember that when the time is right for making love, dressing up prolongs the anticipation and excitement. I love unzipping or unbuttoning a nice tight pair of jeans and stroking the monster raging within through scarlet silk boxers. Slipping your trembling fingers through the gap in his jim-jams doesn't quite have the same effect!

When it comes to dressing up for sex, we girls have got a head start. Let's begin by considering lingerie. Just take a shopping trip to your local high street shops to discover all kinds of scanty, sexy wear. There's matching sets of undies in many different colours, in silks and satins, trimmed with lace; waspies and boned basques to make you look willowy; tasty little teddies that unbutton under the crotch; silky slips and negligées; peep-hole bras; crotchless knickers; and, of course, stockings and suspenders. I know it's a cliché but men really do adore stockings and suspenders. They must have been designed with persuasion in mind. Inform your man you're going to let him fuck you in your best stockings and sussies, and you can literally talk him into anything! Just bring to mind the enticing way the bare belly peeps through between the garter belt and the top of the knickers, and as for that tiny strip of flesh betwixt the stocking tops and the crotch of the panties — well, it's enough to convert any normal chap into a rampant love machine!

And of course there are knickers. There are two things about my knickers that I'm often asked: 'What colour are they?' and 'Can I tear them off?' Knickers in my experience are the flimsy piece of female underwear which provoke male fantasies. A tight little pair of knickers pulled off to one side to reveal an inviting glimpse of pink and allow just enough room to slide in a finger or two, or perhaps a nice stiff prick, is pretty damn exciting, eh?

Knickers come in all shapes and sizes, colours and fabrics. And the panties that we wear often decide our sexual mood. Pretty cotton pink ones for playing at the girl next door. Lacy and white for that virginal feel. Silky, tiny G-strings that cut into our most intimate crevices, and help to keep us wet from noon till night. French high-cut camis that make a girl feel expensive and chic — not forgetting the crotchless ones for days when we are planning a quickie at lunchtime and don't have time to waste!

One occasion when I prefer not to wear any knickers is when I'm out for the evening and dressed in one of my slinky little cocktail numbers. VPL (visible pantie line) is a definite turn off! It's also an incredible thrill to realise that every horny guy who really ogles me is aware that I'm totally naked under my dress. My inspired imagination conjures up a fantasy whereby I sidle off into a dark, private corner and allow a complete stranger to hoist up my dress and explore between my bare thighs. That really gets my juices flowing!

We women feel highly sexual without our panties, but being tucked neatly into our favourite pair of scanties can also feel sensational. G-strings are Polly's elected choice. She tells us exactly why in this letter she sent to me: 'I just had to write and tell you how turned on I get from wearing G-strings. I always used to wear ordinary bikini briefs until a boyfriend bought me a G-string. The following day I put this tiny red G-string on under my skirt and wore it to work. I just felt so randy all day long. Even some of the creeps I work with seemed more attractive! In fact I got a stern telling-off from my boss because I was falling behind with my work. I was supposed to be typing his important letters and there I was with my fingers knuckle deep up my snatch. What makes me so excited is that tiny strip of elastic that I can rub up and down against my clitoris.

'After my boss told me off, I started fantasising that the horny old bastard was going to call me in his office, rip off my G-string and shaft me over his desk. He didn't, but I kept on thinking about it as I carried on playing with my fanny and sucking on my slippery fingers until home time. Now I keep my G-strings out of the office, for fear I get the sack!'

Top glamour model and star of the infamous *Lovers' Guide* video, blonde beauty Marie Harper told me her fancy for knickers: 'My favourite sexual position is doing it doggy and what really makes it exciting for me is doing it with my knickers on. I've got loads of pairs of sexy knickers because being a glamour model, it's a prerequisite of the job. Most of them are minute little pairs that hardly cover my pubes. I prefer older men and I love outdoor sex. I'm not really an exhibitionist, but I like him to slide his hand up my dress, bend me over, whip my knickers off to one side and give it to me hard and fast.'

I asked two twin brothers about their preference in ladies' knickers. Troy, twenty-six, and the eldest by about twenty minutes, works as a model. He revealed: 'I love it in the summer when girls don't cover themselves up so much and you see them flashing lots of leg. Every now and then you get just a little peep at their panties. I suppose if I had to choose, I'd say my favourite knickers are made of raw silk, so they're that creamy kind of colour. When I buy a lady underwear as a present I always go for silk. I really get off on rubbing my dick against cool, smooth silk.'

Twin number two, Derek, also a model, revealed: 'I like red for danger, red for go, go, go! I like those French-cut panties that are high on the thigh and make a woman's legs appear to go on for ever. They're nice

97

and roomy, so you can slip a finger or two in the side when she's ready to hot up. I want to see her parade around just wearing her knickers. Put on a show for me, show me a glimpse of her cunt, play with herself, let me rip them off and taste her. Yeah, you can have a lot of fun with a lady in a pair of red panties!'

I'm sure that many sex guides wouldn't consider devoting an entire section to the joys of pantie power, rubber frocks, thigh boots and naughty nurse outfits, all of which I shall be featuring in this chapter on cute and kinky apparel, but from my stage appearances and from the fantasy mail that pours in by the sackful, I've learnt that sexy lingerie, fetish footwear and uniforms really do turn men on.

When I was working as a columnist for *Club International* I did a six-page spread on uniforms. I dressed up as a traffic warden and posed for a photo session in the notorious clamp zone of Kensington High Street. I got some funny looks whilst straddling my illegally parked Mini Metro with my short skirt pulled halfway up around my arse! I wonder how many of you would love to get hold of a traffic warden, put them over your knee and give them a good spanking. I know I would!

Next I was a sexy schoolgirl decked out in a tiny gymslip and sucking on an enormous lollipop. I even posed on the steps of Harrow Road police station as a miniskirted WPC. That specific photograph prompted many requests for improper use of a police truncheon.

Another uniform that went down well with the men's magazine clientele was a French maid's costume — a teensy-weensy number with a minuscule, circular skirt that accentuated the curve of my arse and revealed plenty of thigh and stocking top. Worn with a lace-front bodice that afforded a good eyeful of cleavage, it looked pretty raunchy.

I remember the night I first wore the maid's uniform. It was some years ago now when I was working for the evening as a personality hostess at this rich guy's birthday party. He had about half a dozen models, all dressed up as French maids, who were there to serve champagne and generally mingle with the star-spangled guests. It's always a problem with these kind of jobs because you get tempted to drink lots of champagne yourself and end up chatting up the hunkiest available man. At this party that was exactly what I did. I suppose it was par for the course, and anyway Birthday Boy wasn't complaining. It was one glass of champagne for a guest and then one for me. Very soon I was a little tiddly and very randy. Champers has that effect on me. I spied this good-looking footballer and we got chatting. He was surprised that I recognised him because, although he's a top player, not many girls take an avid interest in football. I don't either, but I keep a keen eye on the most eligible players!

The party came to an end and people began to drift off home. World Cup Willy and I slipped off to his plush Mayfair flat. I didn't bother to change because he kept telling me how he'd like to tear off my frilly French knickers, lift my satin skirt and fuck me all night long! He was as good as his word. As soon as we were in the lift to his apartment he jammed it between two floors (which in normal circumstances would have made me freak out completely!) and proceeded to tear off my frilly knicks in one fell swoop. He fell to his knees and brought me to a beautiful high with his quick darting tongue. Then he unlaced my bodice and slobbered all over my pink nipples while I unzipped him and got accustomed to his cock. We then had a great quickie fuck against the mirrored walls of the lift!

This story of one episode of my sex life illustrates

perfectly just how much fun you can have when you dress up for sex. To keep you both hard at it, why not pop down to your local fancy-dress shop and slip into uniform? Another uniform that might drive your man crazy with passion is that of a naughty nurse: plenty of bed baths for him, but be careful where you stick that cold stethoscope, girls! Try a WREN's uniform — I just love that tight little skirt and I've always found their hats so sexy! He can strip you completely, except for your nylons and headgear, and take you to paradise starboard! How about dressing up as an air hostess? You can wait on him hand and foot and then let him fuck you in the cramped confines of the downstairs loo! Or perhaps you prefer a trip down Memory Lane? Become the perfect lady in pretty period costume, complete with a hand-made, boned corset and directoire knickers. The biggest thrill with this type of attire is the layer upon layer that you have to struggle through until you chance upon some inviting naked flesh.

Talking of corsets, Elisha Scott, a good mate of mine, disclosed how, with the help of a satin corset, she often enjoys one hell of a good fuck to liven up her morning. Model, ex-Penthouse Pet of the Year, and one-time dancer with the notorious American band the Beastie Boys, Elisha confided: 'If I'm not working, my boyfriend pops home from work mid-morning for his "elevenses". I'm usually ready for him, dressed in a lace-up corset, stockings, suspenders, high heels and no knickers. I wait until I hear his car pull up and that's my cue to bend over on all fours in the hallway, my bare arse and open pussy facing him as he comes through the door. We have a great time!'

Perhaps the feminine garment with the longest history of eroticism is the corset. Its main purpose is to diminish the size of the waist and emphasise the contours of the breasts. The corset must be worn laced in nice and tight so it moulds to the body. It can decrease the waist size by up to about four inches. Not only are they pleasing to the eye, but the hugging sensation feels wonderful. We call the modern version of the corset a waspie or a basque. Victorian corsets were made in all lengths, from a corset as tiny as a wide belt to one that reached from the bosom to just above the knee. They are still being produced today by a firm in Brighton called Axfords, run by ex-model Diane Hasnip and her man. Diane informed me that their corsets are available in satin, cotton and PVC, and in a wide selection of colours. Made by hand, they are all boned and back-fastening, and come with and without brassières and suspenders. I think they look cute worn with nothing but silk stockings or, alternatively, with billowing starchy white bloomers. If you fancy dressing the lady in your life in something Victorian, frilly and very sexy, Axfords is just the ticket.

As I said some way back in the chapter, when it comes to dressing up for sex, we girls do have the widest selection of glamorous garb. But of course when we are wriggling in and out of sexy smalls, shiny PVC and alluring uniform, the men in our life attain a great deal of pleasure. Actually I believe men in uniform can be quite a turn-on too. How about a handsome pilot or a Royal Marine? I don't think I fancy a copper or a traffic worden, though – I've met too many power-crazy ones to be turned on by either! I've seen quite a few male strippers in my time and they can be a lot of fun. Their outrageous outfits range from a tartan-clad Rod Stewart lookalike to air-force pilots, cowboys and leather joyboys. I spoke with Bobby Boy, a top strip artiste, and asked him to divulge his secrets of striptease while entertaining a lady at home.

'I know how much a woman's desire is magnified when she's offered a slow build-up. I dim the lights and invite my lady to make herself comfortable on the sofa. I put on some throbbing music. Standing in front of her, just out of arm's reach, I unbutton my shirt very slowly, pulling it out of my jeans. Then I move a little closer and let her run her fingers over my chest and shoulders before returning to my imaginary stage. I unzip my jeans and slide them over my hips, offering her the first glimpse of my backside and the bulge in my black high-cut briefs. I give it a little help with my hands, run my fingers over my cock and let her feel it through the smooth cotton. Most of my girlfriends become uncontrollable at this stage, so that's the end of the striptease, the beginning of lovemaking.'

An item of essential clothing for a male stripper is the G-string — I find loads of beautiful bare bum, and the way they manage to cram their entire genitals into one tiny triangle of fabric, rather stirring. Another outfit that I find particularly attractive on my men are cycling shorts — Linford Christie is the man we have to thank for bringing those to our attention. So fellas, even if you are two inches short of Linford's personal best, believe me, we girls would love to see you wearing them!

A chapter on sexy clothing would not be complete without mentioning the miniskirt. Since the sixties, men have lusted after long, lean legs flashed from beneath short, tight skirts. I bet there isn't a fella reading this book that hasn't savoured the joys of slipping a warm hand the short distance from the hemline to the pantieline! And we mustn't forget hotpants, another delightful creation from the sixties that are still with us. These days, skin-tight denim shorts that fray off halfway across the bare buttocks are every naughty boy's ideal.

Rubber, PVC and leatherwear offer us a vast array of clobber to titillate; from thigh-length PVC boots to rubber suspender belts and leather chaps, the list of erotic garments in this area is enormous. Many of the PVC, rubber and leather fashions are available in extremely large sizes to cater for transvestites and transexual customers. But aside from cross-dressers, there are many liberated ladies and gents who like to mix fetish clothing with street clothing.

Tina Shaw, a model, striptease artiste and bellydancer, has just opened a new boutique in Camden, north London. She told me about the nightlife fashions on sale at Libido Limited: 'Our clothes are individual because we stock a lot of one-offs from brand-new and established designers. The fashions we specialise in are daring, outrageous and fun. Our range covers items such as a beaded bustier, PVC shorts, lined rubber dresses and a Lycra, rubber-panelled dress. Our prices start at just over a tenner, and rise to two hundred pounds for that special designer outfit.'

I like the idea of a lined rubber dress because, although I adore the look of rubber, I'm not so keen on the way it sticks to my naked flesh. I'm told, however, by Tina, who is somewhat of a connoisseur of rubberwear, that the feel and the smell of the rubber is what appeals to many of her customers. These days rubber fashions have moved a long way from plain black that needs buffing with silicone to achieve that highly polished finish. London designer Kim West now produces sensational rubber fashionwear. In her mail-order catalogue she has on offer a leopardskin-print rubber playsuit, and a slinky leopardskin halter dress, glamorous gold rubber dresses cut low at the back and slit almost to the thigh, and even rubber jackets trimmed with boa feathers at the collar and cuffs.

Leatherwear and PVC provide a comfortable and sexy alternative to rubber. Studded leather jackets worn with lace-up leather trousers look great on well-built men with masses of wild hair that tumbles halfway down their backs. Well, that's my type anyway! We girls look pretty hot in leather too. Leather minis teamed up with a glittery bra top and staggeringly high-heeled PVC thigh boots or shoes will get the bulge in his pants pulsating. I've listed ten items I would recommend women include in their wardrobe. I promise you they'll put the zip back into your sex life and make dressing up for sex more fun than you ever dreamt!

- Pop along to your nearest department store and pick up one of those sexy, silky slips that are now back in fashion. The mini underslips feature delicate shoulder straps and are available in some beautiful colours. They feel fabulous next to the skin, especially when you wear yours wriggled up around your waist for lovemaking.
- A G-string is a must. You've read how horny it makes Polly feel – see what it can do for you!
- Treat yourself to a uniform. Ask him his particular fancy and then buy, hire or make it.
- A matching set of bra, briefs and suspender belt to be worn with sheer silk stockings and high heels. If you can locate a see-through set, you'll drive him wild! You can pick up great, inexpensive lingerie at department stores. If you can't find your favourite colour, buy white and dye the undies to your chosen shade.
- Make your waistline four inches smaller by lacing yourself into a Victorian corset, or perhaps a waspie or basque.
- Flash your lovely legs in a miniskirt. Be confident;

if you don't think your legs are that lovely, just adjust the hemline of an existing skirt by a few inches. I suspect the man in your life will notice the difference.

- Tie-side panties are great for slipping off to one side for some impromptu sex.
- A teddy that unfastens at the crotch is the perfect addition to any sexy lady's wardrobe. Most teddies are quite loose-fitting, so if you haven't got the waistline you desire, who cares! Just let him pop open the buttons between your legs and go to work on your most important button of love.

Well, now you have some idea what kind of exciting attire to get hold of to keep you looking and feeling very sexy, but of course, before we can move on to discuss some interesting locations for testing out all that kinky gear, I'd better assist your shopping expedition by listing where you can buy these titillating garments!

Ann Summers shops sell reasonably priced erotic lingerie for women and some fun G-strings for him. They have four shops: 26 Brewer Street, London W1; 159–163 Charing Cross Road, London WC2; 79 Wardour Street, London W1; and 30 Bond Street, Broadmead, Bristol.

Axfords, established since 1880, make your Victorian dream come true. Delightful corsets, bloomers and accessories are all available mail order. Prices for corsets range from £40–£100 and delivery is within twenty-one days. Their address is Axfords, 82 Centurion Road, Brighton, Sussex, BN1 3LN.

Blunderbuss Antiques sell armour, military uniforms and accessories at 29 Theyer Street, London W1.

Body jewellery is a new range from the **Body Art** people. Dress up your naughty bits by contacting Blake House Studios, Blake End, Rayne, Braintree, Essex.

Hobson De Niro at 27–28 Durham Street, Scarborough, Yorkshire, can cater for all your leather needs, from leather jackets for him to leather G-strings for her.

Kim West's very reasonably priced rubber designs are sold through various shops, but you can buy them mail order from 9a Boundary Road, London E2.

Libido Limited is where you'll find something hot for that special night on the town. You can consult the experts, Tina Shaw and her partner, Debbie Pickford, at 84 Parkway, Camden, London.

She an' Me at 123 Hammersmith Road, Hammersmith, London W14, offers PVC galore, including some outrageous high-heeled shoes and thigh-length kinky boots.

LET'S RECAP!

- 'Inform your man that you're going to let him fuck you in your best stockings and sussies, and you can literally talk him into anything!'
- 'There are two things about my knickers that I am often asked: "What colour are they?" and "Can I tear them off?" '
- 'My inspired imagination conjures up a fantasy whereby I sidle off into a dark, private corner and allow a complete stranger to explore between my bare thighs. That really gets my juices flowing!'
- 'I want to see her parade around just wearing her knickers. Put on a show for me, show me a glimpse of her cunt, play with herself, let me rip them off and taste her. Yeah, you can have a lot of fun with a lady in a pair of red panties!'
- 'How about dressing up as an air hostess? You can wait on him hand and foot and then let him fuck you in the cramped confines of the downstairs loo!'
- 'Within a few seconds of being in your abode, it's trousers down, tackle out, let's fill up that damp pussy with something good, solid and meaty!'

8

Sex in Unusual Places

Making love is a truly sensual experience, and by varying the locations you select for your lovemaking sessions, you can enhance and improve your sex life. Where you make love is as important as when you make love. If you choose an unusual setting for love, not only will your vital erogenous zones be stimulated, but your sense of sight, smell and hearing can be erotically activated as well.

As I've said before, sex in the bedroom can be wonderful. Sometimes there is nothing better than thrashing around on a king-size bed or plunging between the crisp linen sheets with the partner of your dreams. But every now and again, making love elsewhere can put a new lease of lust into your love life. Fucking her on the back seat of your car, or shafting her whilst locked in the stationery cupboard at the office party might be rushed and uncomfortable, but the excitement of leaping on the moment and screwing because you both want it then and there gives the occasion an added sweetness. One thing I've learnt that men find incredibly attractive in a woman is her readiness for sex games where and whenever the mood grips you. The image of taking a willing woman in an unlikely spot plays a part in every male fantasy. I'm not advocating you act like a complete whore, girls, and suggest a fuck whatever the circumstances, but just let him know when and where you want him.

Whilst working as editor of *Penthouse* magazine, my mailbag was often filled with torrid tales of spontaneous and premeditated sexual encounters in various venues. Some of the writers of these explicit letters were so surprised by the excitement and the intensity of their coupling that they seemed compelled to get it down in print and send it off to me. Here's a couple of fine examples:

M.R. of Kent wrote:

For some years now I've had an obsession about screwing girls in cars. It doesn't have to be the exotic model-type creature spreadeagled over the front of my Ferrari — that could never be because I don't own one, and unfortunately don't attract the top-echelon type crumpet portrayed in the likes of girlie magazines — but nevertheless over the last few years I've had some unbelievable sex in my cars. I'm a very safe driver even though I have been known on numerous occasions to savour the sensation of fingering a woman while poodling along the motorway. One such memorable screwing session started exactly like that . . .

Driving along the notorious M25 on the way home from a nightclub, I just knew my date was dying for it. I'd taken her out only twice, and never before had I laid a finger on her, but I knew! We'd only been travelling for a few miles when she eased her bottom back in the seat and propped both legs on the dashboard. I told her to open her legs and she immediately complied. When I slid my fingers beneath her tight, white minidress, she was a little hesitant at first, but when I made contact with her skimpy panties and started to stroke her just where I hoped her clit would be, she moaned and opened her legs even wider. I told her to take off her panties and she couldn't get them off quick enough. I couldn't wait to sink three fingers in that hot twat of hers. What particularly turned me on about this lady, apart from the fact that she had legs that just went on and on for ever, was that she insisted on turning on the interior light of the car, so she could watch my fingers squelch in and out of her cunt. Eyes riveted to her sex, she even used her fingers to pull her pussy lips back, so as to get a good look at my thumb working on her clit. I knew she was going to give me one hell of a time when she took my fingers out and started sucking on them greedily.

My fingers alternating between her pussy and her mouth, I drove off the motorway on to a slip road, and parked up in the first lay-by I came across. If she'd have turned me down at that point, I would have simply wanted to explode. She didn't though; she wanted it just as much as I did. Seconds later I pushed back her seat, wriggled my trousers round my ankles and squeezed into the footwell in front of her. Once in position I slid my hot dick into her with ease. She felt as good as she looked. As I entered her she was still moaning and squirming, still coming from the fingering I'd given her. Her long, slender legs wrapped around me and her tight pussy clenched my dick and squeezed out every last drop of come.

The fact that these two rampant lovebirds were sampling each other's delicious wares for the very first time obviously heightened the pleasures of love in an unusual locale. But couples who have been hard at it

110

for years still enjoy a sexual liaison in weird and wonderful places. Ken from Manchester wrote:

My wife and I adore outdoor sex. At every given opportunity we set off for a day in the country with a mind to fuck *au naturel*! My wife Jean is a very game lass. She's just celebrated her fortieth birthday. I reckon life begins at forty, because at present she's randier than ever. She's a very attractive woman, really full bodied and well preserved like a good wine. She has the most adorable tits I've ever laid eyes on, with huge brown nipples that spring to life with only the merest touch.

It was years ago on a camping holiday in the Lake District that we discovered our mutual love for shagging out of doors. One cool but gloriously bright day, we set off all wrapped up to do a little hiking. We'd only managed a mile or two of our fell walk when it started to absolutely pour down with rain. We found this kind of sheltered archway and huddled together to keep dry. I told you about my missus and her wonderful tits — well, being close to these marvellous mammaries for a minute or two, even in the rain, really made me rampant. Pretty soon, in all winds and weathers, I was sucking hungrily on her sweet nipples.

Now Jean is a girl who really loves her tits to be sucked and after five minutes or so, when her beautiful buds were sticking out like chapel hat pegs, she slid one hand inside my trousers. My cock was really stiff and ready, so I bent Jean over and with her arse towards me and her hands clinging on to the wall, I shoved my manhood between her sticky lips.

That was the first of many. Rarely a picnic goes

by when we don't find a secluded spot to indulge in a smashing outdoor shag. If there are too many people nearby, we always manage to frig each other to a climax.

If I was to bring to mind all the out-of-the-ordinary settings that I've used for carnal couplings, this chapter might be somewhat long, so I've just selected a choice couple that you might find interesting.

It was a glorious summer's day when my boyfriend and I were out walking my three dogs in a cemetery in West London. The graveyard was split up into two separate areas — one section full of ancient tombs and graves, and the other, grassed over, dotted with benches and magnificent trees. Naturally the latter part was fairly full of people enjoying the sunshine.

My man and I chose a slightly secluded spot at the edge of the dead zone. My dogs were running off, sniffing around and amusing themselves, so we sat down under a tree for a cuddle. The cuddling speedily progressed to necking. Then up popped his erection. He's a very big boy and within a matter of minutes it was peeping out of the waistband of his shorts. Now I too was becoming very aroused, so we snuggled ourselves together, and somehow or other we managed to slip his dick up the leg of my shorts to enjoy a lovely fuck spoon-style. We didn't go unobserved, though. As he slapped it into me time after time, I became vaguely aware that we were being watched by the grounds caretaker who was busily cutting the grass whilst riding on a sit-on, power-driven mower.

When we finally finished our delicious tumble, I noticed he was still circling us, and obviously engrossed in our humping, he had been a little over-zealous in his task — the area of grass that surrounded us was cut down almost to the bare soil!

112

Another amusing and immensely pleasurable fuck took place while bent over the loo in a film studio. Going back around ten or eleven years now, I had a small role in a main feature film. I only had a couple of lines, and also I was to perform in a simulated lovemaking scene. Anyway, the director took quite a shine to me and we started going out together. He was incredibly randy and had a very big dick, and in addition to that he was a very nice bloke.

When the movie was almost finished, he called me back to do some voiceovers. When I say voiceovers, I mean those ecstatic, euphoric squeals and gasps that a girl makes when she is bubbling up to orgasm. The director took me into a small studio complete with sound facilities and a large screen. My cameo role was then projected on to the screen. Into a microphone I was instructed to breathe and pant all kinds of sexy, dirty phrases to coincide with the lovemaking scene depicted on the screen. All that grunting and groaning made me as randy as a bitch on heat, and luckily it gave my director the horn too. He made our excuses to the sound engineer and dragged me the few feet to the loo next door, bent me over, tore aside my panties and fucked me very hard indeed. My knickers were naturally somewhat juicy from sex, so I slipped them off and popped them in the top pocket of my jacket when I left.

That night I had a date with my regular boyfriend and I was still wearing the same jacket. I can't recall exactly what happened, except that we had a row and I started crying. I fished around in my top pocket for a hanky, and I ended up drying my eyes with panties reeking of sex. That took some explaining!

The 'little boys' room' might be so named because of the colossal amount of fucking that seems to go on in these unsalubrious places. I recollect one night I was out at a dinner party in a restaurant. There was about a dozen of us there and my mate had the hots for the bloke sitting next to her. He happened to be on a first date with the girl sitting on the other side of him, but that didn't make the slightest bit of difference to my buddy. Between dessert and coffee, the pair of them disappeared to the loo for a knee-trembler, while I had to spend an uncomfortable twenty minutes chatting to this bloke's new bird!

Another of my rampant friends sampled a stiffy at around 35,000 feet when she joined the mile-high club *en route* to Finland on a modelling job. Not only did she get to shag one of the stewards in the confined space of the loo, her arse resting on the stainless steel sink, her buttocks uncomfortable and cold, but so did the other model she was travelling with. Apparently, after guzzling a fair quantity of the buckshee booze, they got a little tiddly, rather randy and egged each other on to proposition the steward. They even tossed a coin to see who got him first!

All the sexy scenarios that I have written about so far fall into the category of unpremeditated sexual encounters. You know what I mean — when you really need some serious shagging so you seize the opportunity and take your pleasures in the most unlikely locations. What I am suggesting is that in addition to these spontaneous frolics you also plan exciting expeditions of sex. Ken and his missus from Manchester seem to have the right idea. Once the happy couple discovered their penchant for outdoor sex, they began to work at it and now contrive their amusement carefully.

There are few sensations as erotic as making mad passionate love on an exotic moonlit beach or wriggling around in a colourful field of golden yellow rape on a warm summer's day. And of course the possibility that you might be overlooked or caught in the act can

114

be an amazing stimulant, although it may have the reverse effect on some couples — the likelihood of getting stumbled upon by a passer-by may give him the dreaded droop! And sometimes the enforced situation of not being able to relax completely whilst frantically fornicating in an unsecluded place causes us ladies to have difficulty reaching a climax. It doesn't with me, I'm happy to say. Being such an exhibitionist, it generally makes me come quicker and more frequently.

So take my word for it, these premeditated fucks are well worth the effort. But I do advise you to do a fair amount of forward planning. For instance, don't decide you're both feeling horny and set off in the car to find this perfect location for some red-hot sex, because you'll probably end up driving around for hours. You'll both get terribly frustrated, end up rowing or shagging in the motor, and if it's in the middle of the afternoon, you might just come up against the problem of Mr Plod tapping on the window when you're straddling your man on the back seat!

Dogging is the quaint British expression used to describe both the voyeurs and the performers who get their kicks from viewing, or participating in, back-seat bonking which occurs in lovers' lanes and car parks around the country. It originated from taking the dog out for a walk — a perfect excuse to slip out of the house, slink off to a well-known spot for courting couples, and watch the lovers perform. However, it is considered extremely bad etiquette to snoop on unsuspecting couples. Somehow or other the voyeur has to be able to decipher which couples actually get off on being watched! Doesn't sound an easy task to me. Consider all those couples who are indulging in a pre-marital affair — I bet it scares the hell out of them. Personally I don't relish the prospect of spectators while I'm snatching a quickie in the car; I may be an exhibitionist, but the idea of all those beady eyes observing me in a dark country lane just doesn't appeal. If it is something you fancy, I would advise you to keep your doors locked to be on the safe side.

A boyfriend of mine, with whom I've spent many a happy hour copulating in cosy car parks, gave me a helpful little hint to keep all nosy parkers from ruining your steamy car sessions. Before you strip off and get down to it in the motor, smear Windolene all over the insides of your windows. Then you can enjoy yourself completely unobserved, and when you are both sated, a quick rub round with a soft clean cloth and you can drive off home with sparkly clean windows!

To find the ideal private outdoor venue for lovemaking you must keep your eyes open for possible locations whilst on your various travels. Then, when the mood is right and you know exactly where you're heading, you don't waste valuable screwing time. It's advisable to set off for your sexy trip well prepared. Take a couple of soft blankets, perhaps some fruit, bottled water, a bottle of wine or even a flask of coffee. All these preparations might seem like a bit of a palaver, but I assure you the end result is worth it. These days we all seem to lock ourselves away in our own private domain and hardly venture into the great outdoors, but the delight of the wind whistling through your hair and your knickers, and being semi-naked in the great outdoors, can be truly wondrous.

Even when you do chance upon that perfect place for love, things can go wrong. A few years ago I was visiting Italy along with my friend, Marie Harper. We were there on a modelling assignment and Marie got her boyfriend to pop over halfway through the trip to spend a few days with her. We both had the day off and were sunbathing around the pool at a private villa set in some spectacular grounds when George, Marie's man, arrived. The lovers immediately sloped off into the bushes for some sex. A few minutes later I heard an agonising scream which sounded very much like one of pain, not of pleasure. And it was — no sooner had George flipped out his dicky than a wasp had perched on the end of it and stung him. Ouch! Perhaps you should include a tube of insect repellant in your list of requirements for your naughty day out?

When it comes to making love in different and multifarious surroundings, it is often the woman who must take the initiative. If the man in your life is a bit reluctant, do your very best to persuade him. Some guys can get a little set in their ways, so I'm relying on you women to talk him round. Think about it, girls, doesn't he usually make most of the running? When you fuck in bed, in the bath, or on the living-room floor, who is it usually makes the first move? My guess is it's your fella.

Be creative about where and when you have sex. Don't be afraid to take the upper hand. Contrive situations that will give your love life that extra bit of spice. Go out on a date, and halfway through the evening, spread your legs and reveal that you're not wearing any knickers. Pop down to his works and swan into his office in your overcoat. Unfasten a few buttons to show him that you're wearing only stockings and suspenders and your tiniest pair of panties. When you are out visiting friends or your in-laws, insist that he accompanies you to the bathroom so he can bend you over the bath and bang you. It's all the more fun because both of you must stifle your screams of pleasure! Or alternatively, wait until he arrives home and be ready for him. Sit astride the kitchen work surface with your crotch thrust forward and your legs well spread. Play with yourself as he walks through the door and asks you what's for dinner. Fuck your way around your home. If you've a sturdy dining table, that can be great fun. The bath and shower are great favourites of mine, as is doing it doggy-fashion halfway up the stairs.

This letter that I received from Rosemary tells a rather interesting tale of how she took the upper hand and demanded sex when she and her husband went round to his boss's house for dinner:

My husband is always trying to climb the promotion ladder. He works in finance and although he had a relatively good job, he still has a fair way to go to reach the top. His boss seems to put him through the paces, and when he invited us over for dinner with him and his wife one evening, my husband Ralph was a little nervous. Gordon, his boss, is a very distinguished gent in his early fifties. I'd a notion that he has an eye for the pretty ladies, and as I'm an attractive, bubbly blonde in my late twenties, I thought I'd dress up in a sexy, low-cut dress to keep the boss sweet. Ralph wasn't sure it was such a good idea, but he didn't push the point.

There were just the four of us at dinner and everything was moving along splendidly. Gordon admired my outfit and gave my slender legs an appreciative glance. He even gave me a big hug when we arrived; his wife Sheila was just checking the dinner at the time. Anyway, the two men sat down on the sofa side by side to talk business, and I sat across from them sipping my sherry. Sheila was still busy in the kitchen and insisted that she should be left alone to get on with it. As the two men chatted, I purposely crossed and uncrossed my legs. My sheer nylons rustled together invitingly. Gordon was not oblivious to my charms and from time to time, in mid-conversation, he'd glance up at me and give me a pleasant smile.

When Gordon popped to the kitchen to see how dinner was coming along, I switched seats and sat next to my husband. It was then that I told him that I didn't have any pants on! Poor Ralph nearly had a funny turn, but he had to cover his embarrassment because it was at this point that Gordon came back in the room to announce that dinner was served.

All through the starter and the main course, I played games with both men. I suppose a couple of sherries and a glass or two of wine put me in that wicked kind of mood. I slipped off my shoes and played footsie with Gordon. At first he was a little timid, but then he responded by moving one leg towards me, enabling my bare, stockinged foot to wriggle right up inside his trouser leg. Still at play with Gordon, I reached out one hand and let it lay dormant on Ralph's fly-button. He gave me a wide-eyed look but didn't remove my hand. I could feel his prick growing hard from my touch.

The meal was first class, but I didn't eat that much. I wasn't particularly hungry, but I was horny. When Gordon and Sheila cleared away the dinner plates and went off to the kitchen to prepare for dessert, I whispered to my husband that I wanted him to fuck me in the bathroom. He shook his head emphatically, so I squeezed his dick a little harder through his trousers and warned him that if he didn't pop upstairs with me to give me a good banging, I'd take his prick out during dessert!

He called out to Gordon that he was just taking me up to the bathroom as I couldn't remember where it was, and we hurried off upstairs. I locked the bathroom door and released his prick, sank down to my knees and gave it a good lapping with my tongue. Now my Ralph usually makes a lot of loud grunts and groans when I suck him, but this time, his lips were sealed!

When his prick was fully hard, he sat down on the edge of the bath and I sat on his lap. He undid the buttons on the front of my dress and massaged my tits as I slowly lowered myself on to his prick. I wriggled around on his prick, desperate to scream out as he grabbed me at the waist and jerked me up and down his length. In more usual circumstances I take a while to climax, but the idea that we had sneaked off from the dinner table to fuck made me very aroused indeed, and I was creaming in only a few minutes, exactly as Ralph shot his hot spunk right up inside me.

When we returned to the dining room the raspberry pavlova was ready and waiting. I'm convinced Sheila had no idea what we had been up to, but I'm sure Gordon knew. It didn't harm Ralph's prospects at all, because two weeks later he advanced one more rung up the ladder.

Some women would probably accuse me of advocating that we become some kind of sex toy, but I dispute that. What I am putting forward is the idea that we as women can decide when and where we make love. If you're not in the mood, he'll have to make do with beans on toast for his tea, not a sumptuous portion of horn on the hob. But when we want it, we should play our erotic games and enjoy our sexual relationships to the full. Sex is only one part of the complicated equation that makes for a stable, happy partnership, but without it many marriages and relationships crumble. If both partners attempt to keep the zing in their love life by regarding lovemaking as a special event that takes time and planning (not forgetting those sudden, uncontrollable lustful urges we all know and love), that will go a long way towards achieving a happy, loving partnership. And we can go on making ecstatic, orgasmic love to the same person for years and years. Or, if you're footloose and fancy free and are well stocked with condoms, you can have a hell of a time as well!

LET'S RECAP!

- 'The image of taking a willing woman in an unlikely spot plays a part in every male fantasy.'
- 'I'm a very safe driver even though I have been known on numerous occasions to savour the sensation of fingering a woman while poodling along the motorway.'
- 'She's a very attractive woman, really full bodied and well preserved like a good wine. She has the most adorable tits I've ever laid eyes on, with huge brown nipples that spring to life with only the merest touch.'
- 'I fished around in my top pocket for a hanky, and ended up drying my eyes with panties reeking of sex.'
- 'Sit astride the kitchen work surface with your crotch thrust forward and your legs well spread. Play with yourself as he walks through the door and asks you what's for dinner.'
- 'I squeezed his dick a little harder through his trousers and warned him that if he didn't pop upstairs with me to give me a good banging, I'd take his prick out during dessert!'

9

Fulfilling Our Fantasies

As the editor of *Penthouse* magazine for several years, I was inundated with fantasy mail, most of it from men who would like to make mad, passionate love to me in numerous ways and forms. But I also receive a great deal of correspondence from sexually aware women whose fantasies, as you can imagine, are not always the same as the men's! The erotic dreams of the ladies often feature frantic lovemaking sessions with their favourite movie star, or perhaps a wish to make love to another woman or experience sex with a stranger – a handsome young delivery boy for instance. But often they want just to persuade their partner to indulge in an unusual sex game.

Each and every one of us has erotic fantasies, and some of these fantasies remain in the brain where they are conceived, acting almost as a pleasure button to activate every time we are alone and feeling sexy. Other fantasies are far more compelling and they become the sex games that we play and enjoy, often affecting the way we make love.

Naturally when we want to act out one of these sexual fantasies, we have to have a willing partner. So what happens when your lover suggests that you do a little role-playing or indulge in something bizarre in the bedroom? Perhaps he'd just like her to dress up as a nurse, or she'd like him to spank her bottom, or wants to eat a ring doughnut off his penis! Well, it's up to you both to decide if you want to participate and indulge in each other's sexual fantasies. And of course, girls, after you've administered all his medicines with loving care, munched that sugary doughnut off his dick or had your bottom turned pink by the force of his hands, with luck the pair of you will be so sexually aroused that not only will you have a delightful sexual coupling, you'll both be in such an intoxicated state of mind that you can make a deal to try out even more of your favourite fantasies.

If, on the other hand, your lover's fantasies seem to you to go too far, you must explain your feelings on the matter. But I suspect if you have discussed your sexual likes and dislikes freely with your partner on other occasions, you would already be aware if he or she had any sexual deviations that you find disturbing. Some you might find unusual, even ridiculous, but, as I've said before, sex is fun and is to be experimented with, so think on before you dismiss your partner's wildest dreams without a second thought.

Here is a letter from Duncan, whose girlfriend is not prepared to indulge him in his fantasies: 'I am twenty-seven years old and have been with my girlfriend for four years now. We are happy together and our sex life is good except for two things. The first problem is oral sex. I very much enjoy having my cock sucked – in fact I often fantasize, Linzi, that your gorgeous lips are gently kissing the tip of my stiff penis. Then your mouth slips down slowly over the head and down the shaft of my by now rock-hard cock. You gently lick and suck until I am unable to contain myself any longer and my spunk spurts into your waiting mouth. My only problem is that my girlfriend doesn't enjoy such pleasures, so I have to content myself with fantasies such as these. The other problem is stockings and suspenders. My girfriend refuses to wear them, saying she finds them uncomfortable, but as I find them an extreme turn-on, I am again left feeling frustrated.'

I received this letter some time ago and I often wonder if he is still with the same partner.

This letter from Simon from east London shows the other side of fantasy. Simon was extremely encouraging and helpful when it came to fulfilling his girlfriend's lesbian fantasy.

My girlfriend and I have an immensely pleasing sex life. We are both open-minded about sex and occasionally have other partners without ill feelings whatsoever. Recently Sarah had been telling me that her ultimate fantasy is to make it with another woman. The idea turned me on a great deal and I was only too pleased to let her have her fun. Nice too, if she'd let me hide away somewhere nearby so I could watch.

The problem of course was to find Sarah a willing sex partner for her first lesbian experience. Strangely enough, it happened when we spotted an ad in the back of a girlie magazine for models. Now Sarah is a very good-looking girl, but modelling seems never to have crossed her mind. She actually works in computers. Anyway, what particularly attracted her attention to this advertisement was its reference to two girls modelling together. We telephoned the number and Sarah was told to go along to an address in West London.

I drove her down there in the car and waited in a side street while she went in for her appointment.

She returned about twenty-five minutes later grinning broadly, telling me that she had the job and had met the girl she was to pose with. I could see that Sarah was excited. As she got into the car, she started to describe the other model. She told me she was just eighteen, had shoulder-length blonde hair, big, firm tits and shapely long legs. Very quickly Sarah became aroused and she demanded that I make her come. I reached over to her and moved my hand up her miniskirt to her inner thigh. Her juices were halfway down her legs already. It took me seconds to push all four fingers in her and I manipulated her clit with my thumb whilst I moved my fingers in and out.

Sarah could hardly wait for Saturday and her modelling job. She asked the photographer whether I could go along if I stayed unobtrusively in the background. I was delighted, but rather surprised when he agreed. I took up my place at the back of the studio and watched them all go to work. The two girls started off in underwear with Sarah reclining on an emerald-green chaise longue. The other model, Louisa, sat on the floor beside her in black lacy undies. The first few shots were of the girls looking at each other. Then it moved on to Louisa reaching up to Sarah's white bra, to take her lovely tits out. She knelt up arching her back as she took Sarah's red nipples in her mouth, moving off to one side slightly so that the camera could catch it all. Sarah's eyes were closed as Louisa's tongue licked wildly all over her nipples. Louisa slid her hand into Sarah's silky panties and I could hear my little baby moaning with delight.

Soon the girls were stripped to stockings, garter belts and their high-heeled shoes. Sarah was laid on her back with both legs high in the air as Louisa knelt over the end of the chaise, pulling Sarah's cunt wide open with both hands and sticking her pink tongue right in.

After the session, Sarah informed me that she had come six times that afternoon. We both went home and went straight to bed, and re-living the session, we made love for hours.

I printed that letter in its entirety because I found it a turn-on, and because it's a prime example of a sexually liberated couple making the most out of fantasy. That particular photo-shoot will keep popping up in their imagination for many sex sessions to come. It doesn't really matter if, when Simon sticks his tongue inside his girlfriend's honeypot, she imagines that his tongue belongs to a sexy model who once tasted her. It is the total experience of sexual fulfilment that is important. And with this particular situation, everyone seems to have had a good time.

Another letter from my mailbag concerns just the kind of role-playing that couples accept to improve their sex lives. Natalie of Leicester writes:

My husband Andrew and I enjoy reading erotic magazines, and find them an enjoyable addition to our sex life. I'd like to tell you about Andy's way with words, which I absolutely adore. He is able, just by talking erotically, to stimulate spasms of sexual excitement in me. He is also your biggest fan, and it doesn't take long for him to be aroused by just seeing a photo of you in a magazine. During lovemaking once, he decided to describe you, in his usual silver tongue, to begin my arousal — and oh, what a turn-on it was! It went like this:

'Linzi's big green eyes stared down at me,

inviting and friendly, her full mouth with large sensuous lips pouted, a girl well aware of her sexuality – I like that. Her long blonde locks, which tumbled in cascades over her shoulders, fell irresistibly over her pert, rounded breasts. Her nipples had noticeably hardened, and were firm to the touch. Her experienced hands with well-manicured red nails slid into her panties, and she lingeringly slipped her silky red French knickers over her tight and beautifully rounded arse. From behind, her never-ending legs ran naturally into her slender, curving hips. Between her playfully spread thighs, you could see a covering of pubic hair, which tapered into the middle of her arse and which bristled with excitement. As she turned, she revealed her Mount of Venus, the heart of her femininity, a goddess before my eyes. The Throne of Love was thickly covered with fine, golden pubic hair, as luxuriant as that on her head. She reached down and artfully spread the hair apart to display the entrance to the magic grotto, with only her lips barring the way to the inner sanctum. Her pussy looked warm and receptive. It was also now moist with her love juices, and heady with her sexual aroma. Beneath her pussy one could delve deeper into her secrets. There, dangling temptingly, was her luscious clitoris – her love button – just asking to be pressed. After fingering, sucking, fawning and nibbling, it would stimulate within her primitive, animal lust, an expression of ecstasy on her lovely face, and her wonderful tits swaying in her delirium. To be one with this personification of womanhood, as both of us merged, and an unrivalled orgasm tore through our entwined bodies, was pure excitement.'

This fantasy was spoken in a slow, rhythmic, but very horny voice. I'm not even into girls, but this erotica flicked my switch, and so, Linzi, you probably see why it had such an electrifying effect on me. I just wanted to feel his length inside, as I couldn't bear it any longer. He gently lowered himself on to me, until just his cockhead was touching my wetness. 'If you want it,' he said, 'take it.' I needed no invitation, and I guided him into my pulsating pussy. As he slid his now throbbing cock deep into me, I was panting like a mare on heat. He began slowly, by stroking fully, and then he began to pump harder and harder, his cock swelling all the time. My orgasmic screams triggered off his climax, causing his hot come to shoot deep in my hole. We were both racked by a climax of sexual excitement, and collapsed breathlessly on the bed. We then shared long, loving 'passion kisses', and both of us groaned with pure ecstasy, thanks to our mind-blowing lovemaking.

Natalie is certainly one lady who appreciates a fantasy for exactly what it is! She obviously knows and loves her man, and is confident enough of her own sexuality not to feel challenged when her lover becomes stimulated by photographs, be they of me or another.

I am always interested to talk to women on the subject of their sexual fantasies. Recently I spent some time in California interviewing XXX-rated movie stars. Naturally I wanted to know their sexual fantasies. Here are some of the responses.

Paula Price, a buxom brunette who has just turned twenty and is nicknamed 'The Anal Queen', told me: 'I can't tell you my fantasy, it's weird. Oh I don't care! My fantasy is to see my husband Eric being fucked by another guy. Actually we were talking about it the other day, and I told him. Eric asked me if I wanted to fulfil it, and I just told him no, let's just leave it as a fantasy!'

Rachel Ryan, a porno actress you might be familiar with from her revelations in the Sunday tabloids (her lovers allegedly include Michael Keaton and Jack Nicholson), told me: 'I have this recurring dream about a quiet, sophisticated kind of man. I fantasise about being with him some place in Europe, somewhere in Florence in an old stone château, with rainstorms and thunder, ice-cool sheets and a hot, smooth man.'

Veteran blue-movie star Sharon Mitchell revealed: 'I think I've acted out just about everybody else's! I've had fantasies just from being with incredibly beautiful women to lots of sadomasochism. That's terrific for me, because I manage to get out a lot of aggression that way. Actually I've just thought of a very funny story about me fulfilling somebody else's fantasy. When I started in the business, I would go and see every movie I'd made. I'd sit there in the theatre and see my pussy sixteen feet high on the silver screen, just like it fucking should be, and that was very exciting. One time, I noticed this terribly good-looking gentleman in the front row and he was slightly grey, but real cute, and he was jacking off, and I was sucking cock on screen. Then I thought, wouldn't it be a fucking mindblower to start sucking his cock and see what he does. So I did! He looked up at the screen, then down at me, then up at the screen again. I was doing exactly what I was doing on the screen to really blow this guy's mind!'

Bionca, a girl who obviously adores her chosen profession, was happy to tell me about her fantasies: 'I remember masturbating when I was quite young and I thought somebody was watching me. Then I'd come just like that. I still have that fantasy that someone is watching me, that always makes me come. I'm sure that's why I got into movies!'

Marilyn Rose, at nineteeen a newcomer to adult movies, told me: 'My sexual fantasy is to have three or four men fucking me in a bathtub full of bubbles. I guess I should mention it to some director who'll probably arrange it for me!'

Madison, a raven-haired raunch queen, revealed: 'I used to have a fantasy about fucking a black man, but then I married one, so that went out the window. Did you ever see the movie *Against All Odds*? It's a really, really good movie, and in one scene, they're down these Aztec tombs, and they're really hot and dirty and sweaty. It's like a sauna. Inside these tombs they're all so sweaty and grimy, and they're just having the most grungy, dirty sex possible. That's what I wanna do!'

Aside from adult movie stars, I have spoken to many women on the subject of their own personal sexual fantasies, and although most of them love talking about sex, when you ask a woman to reveal her most intimate fantasies, those fantasies are frequently vague and undetailed, often borrowed from an erotic book or favourite movie. Even the sex starlet Madison, who spends a large proportion of her life acting out other people's fantasies, nicked her dirty, grungy, sweaty sex fantasy from a feature film! One girlfriend of mine even told me that she'd love to indulge in fantasy and sex games, as long as she didn't have to come up with the ideas herself! So guys, if your head is filled with wondrous sexual fantasies, perhaps you should suggest them to the lady in your life? You may just have a wilder imagination, and she may just be looking for inspiration!

Sexual fantasy often revolves around the taboo. This explicit conversation I had with an acquaintance, a forty-two-year-old widow called Vera, will illustrate exactly what I mean:

My husband sadly passed away four years ago. Since then, I've not had any kind of sexual encounter, although I do masturbate regularly. However, I ran out of coffee the other day and decided to pop next door to my neighbour's to borrow some.

I walked in through the back entrance as I normally do. There is never any need to knock, Angela's house is always an open one. The sight that confronted me as I made my way to the lounge completely took my breath away. It was Angela's sixteen-year-old son, Paul. He was sitting on the sofa, his eyes transfixed on the television, while holding his enormously long penis in his hand. He was giving it such a good pummelling that he didn't even notice my presence.

On the television was a blue movie. Some guy hung like a horse, not dissimilar to Paul, pumping away with a busty, blonde lovely. You can imagine Paul's embarrassment when he did finally see me standing in the doorway. I still have to titter to myself when I think of the expression on his face as he tried to cram his penis back into his trousers! I tried to ease the situation by telling him that what he was doing was a very normal thing to do, nothing at all to be ashamed of, and that I even did it sometimes. That last statement seemed to have a noticeably relaxing effect on him. He asked me why I had to resort to such methods when I was such an attractive woman who could screw any guy, anytime, any place I liked? Of course, I felt very flattered by that, but also very excited that a sixteen-year-old found me, who was old enough to be his mother, attractive!

We sat and chatted for a while until I asked Paul to excuse me, because I had to use the loo. He smiled at me and asked me if he could come and watch me pee. To my amazement, I told him that he could!

Once in the toilet I took off my dress, knickers and tights, but rather than sit on the toilet, I climbed into the bath so that Paul could get a good view. His eyes were nearly bulging out of his head as once again he took out his massive penis and began to stroke himself. This was becoming too much for me. My vagina was simply on fire, I just had to touch him, I just had to have him!

Soon I was strewn across Angela's double bed with my legs flying in all directions as Paul pounded his monster penis in me. It had been four long years and his young penis awoke animal desires I'd almost forgotten I had. I raked my fingernails down his back and called out his name as I came again and again.

It won't happen again — well, that's what I've told myself. I have trouble looking Angela in the eye, knowing how I had sex with her son, on her bed. But oh, it was wonderful! And now when I masturbate, Paul is always there pumping away with that lovely big penis!

As with threesomes, or spontaneously seducing your neighbour's son, the thrill of indulging in forbidden fruit is always a tremendous turn-on, as Vera knows only too well. Aside from the taboo element in Vera's encounter, the other stimulating feature is the spontaneity of the sex. Taking your pleasures with a partner, just when and where you both want it, always feels so deliciously decadent. Personally I believe that those taboo fucks and unpremeditated sex sessions are the ones that float around in our mind, kindling our exotic sexual desires merely by reflection, enabling us to become aroused just by tapping into those heady sexual memories.

It may seem unusual but people I hardly know often open up to me and divulge their most intimate sexual secrets. I'm not sure why I'm treated to these tales of frenzied lust but, believe me, I'm always happy to hear them! The young guy who came to fix my dishwasher told me of a particular sexual encounter with his wife that has fuelled their fantasies and perked up their lunchtime liaisons no end:

I came home unexpectedly from work the other day and found my wife elbow deep in soap suds, doing some hand washing. Nothing unusual in that, you might say, but what was unusual was what happened next! Her skirt was hitched up at the back, and I could see part of her lovely round bum, which got me going. I turned her around and pulled the front of her skirt up. Bits of fuzz were sticking out either side of her minuscule panties. I reached down inside her briefs to finger her and was flabbergasted when she started to unzip my flies, still wearing bright yellow rubber gloves, which were very wet and soapy.

I started rotating my finger in her warm wet fanny as she took out my cock and began to wank me with her rubber gloves. It felt weird and wonderful as her slippery fingers moved up and down the length of my tool. She expertly stroked my shaft until she had me good and ready to fuck her. Her cunt was nice and wet, so I spread her lips and with those squelchy gloves she guided me

133

into her moist slit. The sensation of her rubbery fingers as she steered me inside made my cock ready to explode almost immediately.

The combination of her wet cunt and those rubber-clad fingers gripping my balls was too much for me. Thankfully, I sensed her plump cunt lips starting to quiver and we reached our climax together at the kitchen sink!

Now I often come home at lunchtime and see if I can catch her in the middle of the washing or the washing-up. The feel of that rubber on my cock is magic. If I don't get a chance to take a lunch break, I'm still a happy man — I just sit there thinking about her yellow rubber gloves!

I think it is very important that you understand your partner's sexual fantasies; if you find them a little bizarre or ridiculous, don't be afraid to discuss them, or even have a good laugh about them. Also, if when you are making love, you find yourself drifting off into the realms of fantasy and you're convinced that it's Mel Gibson you are straddling and embracing into your pulsating pussy, or it's Madonna sucking your dick until your cup runneth over, you must not feel you are cheating on your partner. Perhaps, like Natalie, your lover wouldn't be offended, but if you think they might, just keep it to yourself and savour the experience. After all, even if you are dreaming of some fabulous movie star taking you roughly from behind, or some screen goddess spreading her legs for you, it's your partner who's getting the benefit of your untamed sexual excitement. Use erotica if it makes you both horny. Girls, let your man play at being your master, or even pretend he's a total stranger — whatever turns you both on. Whether you've concocted your very own elaborate fantasy or simply borrowed one from a book or a TV programme, have fun! Remember, lots of pleasure can be obtained from erotic fantasy, and it can transform your sex life into a myriad of magical mystery. And after all, learning to improve your sex life is what this book is all about.

LET'S RECAP!

- 'My fantasy is to see my husband, Eric, being fucked by another guy. Actually we were talking about it the other day, and I told him. Eric asked me if I wanted to fulfil it, and I just told him no, let's just leave it as a fantasy!'

- 'She reached down and artfully spread the hair apart, to display the entrance to her magic grotto, only her lips barring the way to her inner sanctum.'

- 'As he slid his now throbbing cock deep into me, I was panting like a mare on heat.'

- 'I'd sit there in the theatre and see my pussy sixteen feet high on the silver screen, just like it fucking should be, and that was very exciting!'

- 'Once in the toilet I took off my dress, knickers and tights, but rather than sit on the toilet, I climbed into the bath so that Paul could get a good view of me pissing.'

- 'I reached down inside her briefs to finger her and was flabbergasted when she started to unzip my flies, still wearing bright yellow rubber gloves, which were wet and soapy.'

10

Sexual Massage

There are basically two types of massage therapy: one that relaxes you and soothes away the aches and stresses and strains, and the other, that not only makes you feel happy and healthy, but horny as well. In this chapter I shall be concentrating on sexual massage that stimulates all those delicious pleasure points as well as the sexual organs themselves. Now I'm not suggesting you pop down to your local seedy massage parlour to indulge — you might well experience a good hand job or, equally likely, get ripped off. What I am advocating is that you and your chosen partner learn about sexual massage in order to pleasure each other fully.

I have two friends, Nigel Verbeek and Sarah Dale, who are trained in the art of massage. Nigel has kindly given me some assistance with this chapter. You may be familiar with the name Sarah Dale; she is in fact a sex therapist. The *News Of the World* thought otherwise when they concocted a story about Sarah while she was renting a house from Conservative MP Norman Lamont. At one time Sarah and I were embarking on a video project together and we spent some time discussing many sexual subjects, one of which was massage. Sarah confided to me, and I quote: 'When I massage the body, I massage the entire body. That to me is the whole principle of body massage.'

Sounds very reasonable to me, and, no doubt, immensely satisfying, unlike that exclusive 'ladies only' retreat I used to frequent for an occasional massage. Here's a letter I received from Cathryn, who has recently discovered the delights of sexual massage:

My sex life has taken on a new dimension since meeting Neil, a man who is a trained masseur. I always thought that the concept of massage is to relax you completely. Often, when I've had a massage in my local health club, I've dropped off to sleep. But the kind of massage that Neil practises on me definitely does not make me feel sleepy − relaxed and randy as hell, I should say. Let me tell all.

Firstly we dim the lights and put some soft music on the stereo. We prepare the bed and I undress. I lie on my belly and Neil sprinkles my naked body liberally with aromatic oil. Then, in gentle rhythmical movements, he works the oil over my body, paying particular attention to my bottom.

He spreads my legs and begins by lightly scratching my inner thighs. His touch gets lighter and lighter as he approaches my cunt. He reaches up between my legs and cups a hand over my entire pussy. Grabbing a handful of my flesh, he manoeuvres it around. He uses the palm of his hand to squeeze and massage my pussy. By now I beg him to use his fingers. He slowly slides one finger above my clit hood and two inside my pussy. Now he can lovingly caress all the surfaces of my pussy. I'm really hotting up now, so I roll over on to my back.

Neil applies more oil and smoothes it on to my tummy and breasts. He circles my greasy nipples, centering on my areolae but never touching the nipple itself. Of course I want my nipples to be stimulated, so I have to ask. He obliges by brushing his spread fingers over my nipples, every now and then holding my nipple between his thumb and forefinger so they get stimulated and thus lengthen.

With my excitement rising to fever pitch, I implore him to massage my pussy. Once again he uses the palm of his hand to arouse me. Then he parts my lips and runs his forefinger up and down the length of my slit. Generally it is at about this point that I beg for his tongue. My body is tingling from my head to my toes and it feels like my pussy is about to explode if a wet tongue is not inserted very swiftly. It's at this point that massage stops and the dynamic sex begins. Massage is a hell of a form of foreplay!

Cathryn is indeed fortunate to have a trained masseur as the love of her life. But as long as you and your lover are both willing to learn how to pleasure each other in this relaxed, ethereal way, there's every possibility that sexual massage will work for you. Massage is a voyage of discovery for the giver and the taker. Any limits on what you both want to happen should always be set beforehand. You must trust each other implicitly, and if you are practising safe sex, remember to wear medical gloves if you have any cuts or grazes on your fingers or hands.

Before commencing with the massage, you should know what you are doing. The first things to learn are the body's pressure points.

For her these are located from the sternum to the belly-button and beyond to the pubic bone in a straight line; in a 'V' shape either side of the pussy rather like the line of a G-string; down the front of both legs, creeping towards the inner thigh rather than the centre of the leg, from just below the vulva stretching down vertically to just above the knees; and rolling over, the small of the back to the upper part of the buttocks, two straight lines on either side of the spine; at the centre of the top of the head; and at the centre of the base of the skull.

And for him, exactly the same with reference to the head, base of skull, down the legs and around the pelvic region. Rolling him over, his pressure points on the back are similar, but are more concentrated at the base of the spine, the top of the sacrum bones on either side, and on both sides of the crease of the buttocks.

In addition, for both sexes, parts of the soles of the feet are erotic trigger points, as is the big toe and the area a couple of inches either side of the bone running from the back of the heel up towards the calf of the leg.

Now you are aware of the pleasure points you can begin with sensual massage. Firstly undress — if you are in agreement that the massage will act as a prelude to lovemaking, it is advisable that you both strip naked in readiness. Then prepare the room carefully. Clear away items such as work papers or business matters that might prevent you or your lover from relaxing completely. Turn the lights down low and light a few candles; perhaps burn a joss stick or two. Enhance the atmosphere of the room to create the particular aura you both desire. If you intend to perform the massage on the bed, lay out a large soft towel to protect your bedding. If you're giving the massage on the floor, use a couple of blankets beneath the towel for comfort. And of course make sure that the room is warm. It's a good idea to take the phone off the hook so you won't be disturbed. Music is a wonderful accompaniment. Take your pick from classical, gentle music or even heavy rock. Available on the market are audio tapes that feature cascading waterfalls or the sounds of the sea crashing to the shore. All these added extras can heighten your pleasure as you surround yourself with relaxing sounds and aromas.

Use aromatic oils to enhance the erotic sensation that is sexual massage.

FOR HER
Neroli is intensely female, relaxing yet stimulating.
Ylang-ylang is sweet and stimulates the senses, soothing away the frustrations of life.
Clary sage is like a seductive man — it makes you heady and euphoric, and stimulates the sexual woman in you.
Rose maroc is luxurious, earthy and erotically sexual. If you use it, you had better mean it!
Jasmine is powerful and provokes the ultimate image of woman in a man.
Coriander is uplifting, spicy and provocative, and will stimulate you into action.

FOR HIM
Cardamon is spicy and profoundly sexual in nature, evoking sensuous, erotic thinking.
Ambrette is animalistic and stimulates the sexual man.
Bay is distinctive and sexually arrogant. Not for the submissive!
Jasmine is the mistress of the night, bringing out man's desires and fantasies.
Cumin is erotic, bizarre and evocative. It can powerfully stimulate the flow of bodily juices.
Ginger is arousing, inviting and satisfying.

Now the scene is set, lay your recipient face down, eyes closed, their arms cushioning their head, and smooth your chosen oils on their back, buttocks and legs.

140

Become aware of their breathing and begin to breathe in time with them. This builds up a sympathetic energy flow. Throughout the massage maintain continuous hand contact. Never stop the massage procedure abruptly unless specifically requested to do so. Slip into rhythm slowly and surely, so the brain can relax and concentrate solely on the area of the body being massaged. It's a journey of discovery with one pleasurable sensation drifting into another. Once you have finished massaging the back, turn your partner over so you can go to work on the front of their body. Apply more aromatic oils, and remind your partner to keep their eyes closed; you can use an eye mask if you wish.

Let us begin with a basic massage. It is important to know that all massage movements should be relaxed and unhurried. There's plenty of time to move on to sexual zones. The slow build-up will make it all the more pleasurable. Commence with the head. Make sure your hands are free of oil, then explore the pleasure points on the head. Start at the base of the neck and work towards the crown.

When you practise erotic massage there are really half a dozen separate types of technique to use − but note that the aggressive Scandinavian style 'chopping' we see in the movies is not one of them!

Effleurage is stroking. The strokes can be long or short, and these movements are the basic components of sensual massage.

Petrissage uses the whole hand and can be compared to the action of kneading dough. The buttocks respond well to this type of massage.

Vibration is a trembling movement. This action is practised with either the forefinger, middle finger or thumb. The movement is very light and is particularly good for use on the sexy stimulation points.

Acupressure is also used on the pleasure points, pressing with fingers or thumbs to energise the meridian.

Hacking is a light and quick flicking and chopping motion with the edge of the hand.

Plucking is the name given to the technique of working your way towards the pubes, plucking hairs either side of the scrotum or vulva to open things up. This is used as the entrée to sexual massage. We'll leave that just for now because we want to build up to that moment in a leisurely manner.

When beginning to massage the body, put your whole weight behind your movements. Opinions differ on the route that the giver should take. Some like to work their way very slowly down from the neck to the buttocks, and others from the buttocks up to the neck. Both variations take in the pleasure points en route. Aside from that disparity, all the massage professionals I consulted when compiling this chapter agreed that the movements should always be towards the heart and should be approached as follows. Work from the feet up to the buttocks, paying special attention to the erotic trigger points once you have located them. When massaging the arms, start at the hands and travel up to the shoulders. While working on the breast or chest area, you should move upwards towards the neck and outwards towards the shoulders. And finally, massage the stomach with clockwise, circular movements.

The concepts of sexual massage are the same for women and men but the different anatomies need to be described separately.

FOR HER
Spread the legs wide and lightly scratch and trail your fingers along the inner thighs. Lighten your touch as

you approach the labia. Scratch the pubic hair as if you are combing it to groom it. Avoid the sensitive parts and stimulate the skin as you would a scalp. With your index and middle finger, slowly rub from near the anus to just in front of the clitoral hood, along the outside of the lips. Stretch the clitoral hood and the labia, to increase swelling. Use the palm of your hand to massage the entire vulva, gingerly rotating it and sliding over it. Take a handful of flesh with the clit in the middle and gently manoeuvre it around. Using your three middle fingers, do rhythmical rubs and oval circles all over the vulva at a controlled speed. Part the lips and run your finger up both inner thighs to the clitoris, then manipulate the clit hood. Lay her on her stomach and place one finger just above the clit hood and two fingers inside her pussy, the ring finger on the perineum, and the thumb into the anus. Move your hand around, gently at first, feeling your thumb and forefinger rub against each other. Lay her on her back again. Insert a finger and lovingly caress all the surfaces of the vagina.

FOR HIM

Men often prefer talcum powder to massage oil, or alternatively you can just use saliva. Begin once again from the plucking stage during body massage, then scratch up the inner thighs, brushing against the balls and scratching the pubic hair. Pull the balls back to stretch the skin. Take the base of the penis in your hand and grasp it further and further towards the head with tiny massage movements. With a well-lubricated palm glide the flat of the hand across the tip of the penis. Hold the shaft and move the skin up and down it. If he has a foreskin alternate the amount you slide it up and down. You can do this very slowly or exceedingly fast; ask your man which he prefers. Continue with this movement but now use both hands, one to massage the shaft firmly and deeply, the other working in time but in the opposite direction. Hold the foreskin back if he has one and tease the frenulum by making circles with your fingertips and gently stroking it, sometimes trailing your fingers all around the circumference before returning to the frenulum again. If he has a foreskin hold it back and put all your fingers around the head and squeeze the urethra, dwelling there and then starting again. Some men like to have their balls held all the time, while others prefer them to have particular attention paid to them; this can range from squeezing to light peripheral touches.

FOR HIM AND HER
Circle the anus without entering to tease the rim into begging a finger inside. Nipples are very individual, and yet the more you hot up for sex, the more versatile they become. Lightly run fingers around the nipples, centring on the areolae, but never actually making contact with the nipple. Brush spread fingers over the nipple and then grasp them between the thumb and forefinger. If you enjoy heavy manipulation, squeeze the nipple vigorously, twisting it around and pulling it away from the breast. Take the whole breast in your hand and, holding the nipple between the gap in two fingers, squeeze and move it around the chest.

I suspect that you'll find some or most of these massage techniques arousing and fulfilling, and hopefully when practised they'll create enough stimulation to make you both very passionate indeed. Sensual massage heightens sexual vibrancy, sensitivity and response, and when you are both extremely turned on from your massage experience I'm convinced that an ecstatic lovemaking session will take place.

Before I conclude this chapter on sexual massage, I must divulge my tale of an extremely thrilling massage that I encountered while on vacation in Bangkok several years ago. Now downtown Bangkok offers sex for sale in many various forms, but the one sexual pleasure on offer that I could not resist was a sexy massage. I'd heard on good authority that the kind of massage given in Bangkok was unlike any other. Well, I'm the kind of girl who likes to try out new adventures, so along with my travelling companion/boyfriend, Simon, we sought out a massage parlour — and were pleasantly surprised to discover what a grandiose, majestic establishment we'd stumbled upon.

We were ushered into an absolutely vast luxurious reception area, with a huge window all along one side. Ensconced behind this glass partition sat approximately fifty Oriental girls, all dressed in their finest evening attire and sporting a badge with a number on. We quickly realised that this was the viewing area, and that although we could ogle the talent and make our selection by number, the jewels of the Orient on the other side of the window were unable to see the customers.

Over a gin and tonic we paid our money and took our choice. After much deliberation and some recommendations from the proprieter, we chose a delightful beauty in her early twenties called Sue Lee. Although there wasn't a huge demand for it, Sue Lee was very keen on massaging couples, as we were helpfully informed by the owner.

Sue Lee took us off into the massage room, which was a very clean, white tiled room complete with a double bed, an enormous bathtub and a lilo. She handed us both a towel and suggested that we undress.

Together the three of us stripped naked. Sue Lee possessed a darling figure: tiny little hips, a petite waist, a thick batch of black pubic hair and gorgeous pert budlike breasts. I could see Simon's cock stirring almost immediately.

Sue Lee filled the tub and bade the two of us get into the steamy froth. She joined us, and one at a time she washed us all over, her nimble fingers exploring our bodies as she lathered us expertly and erotically.

All clean, we clambered out, and Sue Lee dried us with a fluffy white towel, sprinkled us liberally with talc, and then enquired, in quite good English, which of us would like to be first. As ladies first was the order of the evening, she requested that I lie down on the lilo so she could go to work.

The western concept of massage is that the hands are predominant, but the Thai theory is to forget manipulation with the hands and use the masseuse's entire body! With a bucket of hot, soapy water and a sponge, Sue Lee squeezed bubbles all over my back, buttocks and legs, lathered up the front of her own naked form and, seconds later, straddled me and wriggled her nubile, taut body up and down my slippery, wet one. Her skin felt electric against my sizzling flesh and I began to tingle all over. In a dreamy, euphoric state I glanced up at Simon and noticed his excited expression as he sat naked upon the bed, one hand grasping his erect cock, stroking it steadily, his eyes fixed upon us, enjoying the spectacle.

Time seemed to stand still as this lovely creature climbed all over me. I could feel the hardness of her nipples, the coarseness of her pubic hair and the sensation of her open cunt rubbing enthusiastically against me. Just when I was drifting off into fantasyland, my reverie was broken momentarily as she turned me over to lie on my back. Simon was now wanking furiously. I grinned at him as Sue Lee sank back down on to me, her legs spread, her hairy cunt gaping. Delicate fingers caressed and kneaded my breasts as her slippery body and dripping cunt rode up and down my trembling torso. I was squealing with delirium as the frenetic friction of our shuddering bodies brought about a simultaneous climax for myself and my sexy masseuse.

Before attending the massage parlour, we had made the decision that we would fuck only each other. We would allow Sue Lee to excite us both to fever pitch, and then go on to fuck each other's brains out. We had decided on that outcome because we were keen to practise safe sex.

Now it was Simon's turn for a little piece of Oriental heaven. The poor man had great difficulty lying face down on the lilo because of his massive erection, but we both knew only too well that if he were to lie on his back while Sue Lee worked her tantalising body up and down him, his cock would have certainly slipped inside her hot, hairy hole. So Simon lay face down, carefully adjusted his stiffy and let Sue Lee smother him with her squelchy, alluring nakedness. Reclining on the bed, I squeezed my bulging red nipples and fingered myself as I watched them at it.

Things got hot and sticky then. It was only a matter of minutes before the erotic body massage was abandoned and the three of us were entwined, naked on the bed. Sue Lee and I knelt either side of Simon and sucked and licked at his cock, our tongues working together, flicking and dancing up and down the length of his throbbing shaft, circling his knob and lapping at his balls. In just a few minutes he had splattered us girls with his cream.

Simon's cock hardly decreased in size after he'd shot his load, but while ecstatic tremors were still traversing through his body, Sue Lee used the short impasse to allow me the pleasure of her tongue. With a featherlike touch, she teased the length of my slit, poked inquisitively into my arsehole and then homed in on my clit. It felt sensational and just as I was starting to go into spasms, I felt Simon roll me over on to my knees and slip his hot dick easily inside my pulsating pussy. He grabbed handfuls of my arse cheeks as he pumped his raging cock hard into me, his balls slapping against my quim. Sue Lee wriggled beneath my body, played with my hanging breasts, eagerly feasted on my cunt and, when she had a free hand, gripped on to Simon's piston-like prick.

That was certainly one episode involving sexual massage that Simon and I will never forget!

LET'S RECAP!

- 'He spread my legs and begins by lightly scratching my inner thighs. His touch gets lighter and lighter as he approaches my cunt.'
- 'With a featherlike touch, she teased the length of my slit, poked inquisitively into my arsehole and then homed in on my clit.'
- 'Some men like to have their balls held all the time, while others prefer them to have particular attention; this can range from squeezing to light peripheral touches.'
- 'Circle the anus without entering to tease the rim into begging a finger inside.'
- 'I could feel the hardness of her nipples, the coarseness of her pubic hair and the sensation of her open cunt rubbing enthusiastically against me.'
- 'Our tongues worked together, flicking and dancing up and down the length of his throbbing shaft, circling his knob and lapping at his balls.'

11

Mouthwatering and Messy

I once received a letter from a gentleman whose favourite fantasy was for me to munch a ring doughnut off his dick. Sugary and sweet and very tasty, no doubt! That little gem of correspondence got me ruminating on the connection between two sensuous pleasures — food and sex. Aphrodisiac treats create sexual desire: bananas and cucumbers act as satisfying, surrogate sex toys. Try smothering your lover's genitals with raspberry yoghurt and falling upon the feast to guzzle greedily, or just experience the sheer joy of relaxing with your partner and feeding each other exotic, erotic food. Naughty nibbles can be delightful and delicious.

We can all probably evoke an incident in our sex life that was mouthwatering, yet messy. Phallic foods sliding between glossy painted lips can drive a guy to distraction — take the Cadbury's Flake commercials as a prime example. Glossy red lips gorging on dribbling strawberries, delicate fingertips peeling back the skin of a banana before slowly sliding it between wet, parted lips really turn a man on. I recall one evening when I was out on a first date, eating with my fingers, feeding my man hot, dripping asparagus. Not only did it give him the correct signals, but it made him so charged with sexual energy that he fucked me

149

within moments of leaving the restaurant! Good sex involves much slipperiness and secretions and that is possibly why sticky, gooey food can be such a thrill.

Take a look at this letter I was sent from Cassie, who obviously like to indulge in food frolics.

For some years now, I've had a thing about creamy, sloppy foods like fresh cream, jelly, trifle and custard. Ever since I can remember I've always wanted to be one of those ladies who was hired for special banquets and made to lie on a table and get covered in whipped cream, ice cream and juicy fruits. The ravenous party revellers would lick and suck the delicious stuff from my helpless, edible body.

I've always longed to meet a man with a similar interest, a man who would go crazy at the thought of shoving an ice-cream cornet straight up my snatch, then eating it out. Recently I met just such a man. When I confided my love for messing about with foods, he invited me round for an evening of delicious sex that I'll never forget!

When he led me into his bedroom the bed was already covered in a sheet of black polythene. He told me to strip off and lie on it. While I slipped out of my clothes, he disappeared. By the time he returned holding a jug, I was lying naked on the cool plastic sheeting, stroking my hot snatch.

'Close your eyes,' he ordered and I immediately complied. I felt a warm, wonderful thick blob squelch on to my tits, my belly button, and between my open legs. I didn't know what it was, but it aroused me immensely. 'Open your eyes,' he said, his voice trembling slightly.

I discovered I was smothered in smooth, milky

custard, and I lay there quivering while he licked off every last drop, making absolutely sure that not a sticky drop remained on my hard, jutting nipples, in my navel or around my hairy cunt.

Then he disappeared again and came back with a spray can of whipped cream and a handful of ripe strawberries. He squirted the cool cream in a thick stream from my neck down to my crotch, then strategically placed the strawberries, one on each nipple, one in my belly button and one just below my clitoris. Slowly circling each nipple with his tongue, he devoured the strawberries, then sucked the one from my navel. His cock was huge and swollen and nudged me in the tummy where it became covered with cream. I bent forward, slipped it gently into my mouth and delighted in the sensational taste of sweetness mingled with his juice.

When he lowered his head to tackle the strawberry nestled between my cunt lips I was moaning and squirming, and beside myself with excitement. By now the cream had dribbled into all my crevices and he had set himself the task of running his tongue everywhere, inside and out. I was slithering around on the polythene, feeling wet and sticky all over my arse and back. Then he poised himself above me and lowered himself on to my creamy body. I had the satisfaction of feeling the cream squish and spread between our bodies as he penetrated me.

He fucked me with his cream-covered cock. My tits slithered against his chest as we squirmed about, spreading the goo all over each other. I shuddered in orgasm after orgasm. When he groaned that he was coming, I grasped his cock and pulled it out of me, held it and wanked him furiously. With delight I watched as streams of white spunk splattered all over me and the black plastic. It was the best and messiest fuck of my life!

I have a girlfriend who bravely volunteered to act as the sweets trolley at the 1990 Sex Maniacs' ball. Vietta told me: 'I was wheeled in prostrate on a trolley, my nakedness covered only with fruits, whipped cream and, would you believe, honey! It was certainly an arousing experience having dozens of men and women feasting on my body, not to mention the fumbling fingers that delighted in smearing sticky honey all over and up my cunt!'

Perhaps I'll take Vietta's place at the next Sex Maniacs' Ball? Her tale brings a whole new meaning to the expression 'honeypotting'! I can also identify with Cassie's fresh cream fuck, although I personally don't like to go quite as far.

A few years ago I was offered a small TV role in a drama series. I was to play a belly dancer and perform on a table for a group of rowdy pressmen. After twirling my tassels and stripping out of my skimpy costume, I was bombarded with fresh cream trifle! Funnily enough, only two of the chaps slinging the slop were privy to the scene previously. The other half a dozen or so were extras, who turned up on the day to be informed that their day's work consisted of ogling a stripper, then smothering her in trifle! Fun, eh? But I digress. The point of this anecdote is that I saw my role as fun, but not as a turn-on. Quite frankly I was more concerned with learning the technique of tassel-twirling than with becoming horny from the sensation of being smeared with sherry trifle. But this acting part did have its benefits in the form of the director, whom I found both charming and sexy.

As I was to perform my scene twice, it was obviously necessary to get cleaned up completely in between takes. So, in the morning I did take number one. It was a laugh and the smooth slippery trifle squelching on my breasts and belly felt gorgeous. The director flirted with me and told me I'd done a great job, which prompted me to spend the entire lunch hour in the bath cleansing my important little places, playing with myself, and hoping desperately that the director would be a lovey and come to assist me in my enjoyable clean-up campaign. Unfortunately he didn't, but just lying there in the steamy hot bath, thinking about what might have been, made my second performance even more enjoyable.

I asked a few friends to tell of their mouthwatering, messy experiences:

Kim, an old schoolchum from Bristol, revealed: 'My boyfriend and I are both chocaholics and we like nothing better than mixing our craving for chocolate with our craving for sex. He likes to slide a Mars Bar up my cunt and then lick me out. Sometimes we share the chocolate that becomes soft and gooey and smeared with my sexual juices.'

Trevor has a penchant for fruit: 'My new girlfriend is really highly sexed and just loves to try anything bizzare or unusual. The other night, she suggested that I slide a banana into her pussy. It was delicious, but next time, she says it's best if I warm the banana first, as the coolness of the ripe flesh put her off slightly.'

'Champagne is the perfect aphrodisiac for me,' admitted Vicki, a model from Scotland. 'Just a glass or two makes me really randy. I like to dribble the cold fizz all over my nipples and pubes and get my bloke to lick it off. Sometimes I get the urge to feel the neck of the bottle between the mouth of my minge. I get him to insert it gently, then once it's pushed a little way in, I tell him to shake the bottle carefully and a whoosh of bubbly, frothy liquid shoots right up inside my fanny. Instant climax time!'

One chap wrote to me and told me of an unusual solitary game that gets him off: 'I cut a hole in the top of a water melon, pour in a little hot water, then fuck it. I highly recommend it!'

I keep using quotes from porn star Sharon Mitchell, but I'll make no apologies, because she's one lady who has many interesting things to say on sexual subjects. When I asked her what was the kinkiest sex scene she's performed for the camera, she grinned broadly and answered: 'The weirdest thing that I've ever done on film was to fuck Eric Edwards in a vat of warm spaghetti. All those wriggly bits of pasta squelching around all over my body felt real weird. Personally I didn't think it looked too photogenic, but that's what the producers wanted, and we managed to do it!'

I suppose Sharon and I are both in a profession that calls for us girlies to perform weird and wonderful stunts on occasions. I remember quite vividly sitting, dressed only in a miniscule bikini, in a bathful of custard outside a pub on the Holloway Road, London, on a busy Friday afternoon. I think it was for charity, but goodness only knows why it called for me to exhibit myself in such a strange manner! Mind you, I am quite at home wriggling around in large receptacles filled with sticky, stodgy goo. For instance, I mud-wrestled Penthouse Pet Elisha Scott for the television cameras in one episode of the sitcom *Sorry*, and my debut appearance on video was in an Electric Blue special – a mucky masterpiece entitled *Nude Jello Wrestling*.

I began my performance in the video by strutting around dressed as a sexy schoolma'am selling kisses for a pound a time to a very exuberant audience before stripping out of my outfit to rapturous applause and getting to grips with a scantily clad nurse (in the delightful form of Marie Harper) whilst writhing round in a giant rubber pool filled with strawberry-flavoured jelly!

The audience cheered and the compere ranted on benignly as the mouthwatering Miss Harper and I slid all over the place, ripping off each other's tiny G-strings and bras. As I was rather more buxom that Marie, the contest was supposed to be fixed for me to win, but Marie was a little overawed by the situation and seemed determined to have the upper hand. She transformed herself from the naughty but nice Nurse Harper to a rampaging wild animal, sloshing jelly into my open legs, massaging handfuls of goo into my sticky titties and generally climbing on top of me, straddling me with her naked, slippery body and pinning me down into a hold. In that inflated paddling pool full of wobbly jelly, she manoeuvered me into a compromising position and grunted: 'I'm going to get you to submit!' I didn't object — I was having far too much fun — so I just lay back and let her get on with it. I did get a few good gropes of her jelly-covered arse and tits, of course!

The grande finale to the video was even better. All six girls featured in *Nude Jello Wrestling* clambered back into the pool along with four male volunteers. To us foxy females it seemed rather unfair that we were all starkers and the fellas weren't, so we proceeded to separate the men from their clothing. It was wonderful, a wild orgy of lusty ladies dunked liberally with cold, strawberry jelly, tearing off the guys' gear. They were outnumbered and had no chance!

It's not only jelly that I've wrestled in. I once wrestled three lovely models in a paddling pool of chocolate-flavoured porridge! It was back in my *Club International* days and the porridge was actually due to a technical hitch. I was supposed to be presenting the *Linzi Drew Jelly-Wrestling Extravaganza* – but the bloody jelly wouldn't set. My glamorous mates and I didn't want to be swishing around in this gory red liquid looking like victims of a cheapo thriller movie, so we had to come up with a compromise. One bright spark suggested chocolate-flavoured porridge, and I suppose it could have been worse. Squidging around in porridge was quite pleasant; it smelt delicious and felt soft and warm, kind of like an all-over face pack, but the colour of the stodge was somewhat unfortunate – slightly reminiscent of a giant cowpat! And the other drawback was that it was so thick and mushy that even when we girlies were stark naked, the magazine reader would get short shrift with regard to getting a good glimpse at our bouncing boobies and hairy pussies. We looked rather like four giant gingerbread ladies without a hint of pink pussy in sight!

It didn't turn me on, but I can well see how it excites many lovers of slapstick sex. There are specialist magazines and videos on the market that feature gorgeous gals getting their protuberant parts doused in just about everything from spaghetti to motor oil. Picture the scene: a busty blonde stands in her kitchen stirring a saucepan of custard. A lascivious look comes across her face and then she slowly tips the whole lot down her cleavage. Pretty soon she's joined by another lovely and the pair of them roll around on the kitchen floor covering themselves from head to toe in various substances, all available from your local supermarket! A word of warning here: if you fancy this kind of unusual entertainment and you're not completely sure that your other half will be eager to join you in a splatterfest *extraordinaire*, do broach the subject first before scrunching a black forest gâteau down the front of his or her panties!

On a more sophisticated note, we move on to sensual food and wine. The ancient Chinese appear to have been the first to add perfume to their wine. The Romans perfumed their wines to produce fidelity in love. Of course, wine itself can be an aphrodisiac. The Egyptians, Greeks and Romans all used wine for its aphrodisiac properties, claiming quite correctly that it brings warmth to cold parts. Wine can act as a relaxant and a stimulant. It can loosen you up and help diminish tiresome inhibitions. But too much wine can produce the dreaded droop for him, so make sure he sips moderately.

The word 'honeymoon' derives from the old Saxon honey wine potion that men drank for thirty days after their wedding to improve their lovemaking. One cupful a day was apparently enough! Here's the recipe, along with another couple of exotic, erotic love potions making use of aromatic oils and herbs.

HONEY WINE
1 bottle of white wine
1 tablespoon of clear honey
1 pinch of ground coriander
1 pinch of nutmeg

Warm over a low heat.

LOVE FLIP
Blend together:
1 egg yolk
1 glass of port

½ glass of brandy
1 teaspoon of sugar
1 drop of rosewater

Add crushed ice and serve in your most attractive wine glasses.

Aphrodite's Nectar is a very simple potion to make. It's based on an ancient recipe that is said to give you youthful beauty and increase your sexual appetite!

APHRODITE'S NECTAR
1 bottle of wine (red or white according to preference)
2 pinches of rosemary
2 pinches of sage
4 pinches of cinnamon
4 drops of orange essence
2 dessertspoons of sugar
1 small glass of rum

Mix all the ingredients together and leave to infuse for three days.

Forget all than nonsense about gorging yourself silly on oysters in an attempt to boost your libido — you'll quite likely end up with an upset tummy and no sex drive whatsoever! Give one or all of these ancient, exotic potions a try instead.

Now before I go off and whip up a captivating liquid concoction in my Kenwood, here's a list of foods that I find increase my sexual vibrancy.

CREME BRULÉE
This is a sheer taste sensation, filled to the brim with calories and so deliciously sweet that the mere taste can almost bring me to the point of orgasm.

158

I would recommend you savour this creamy, caramelised dessert in a restaurant, as it's not easy to get the consistency exactly right when making it at home. More importantly, it tastes so much better if you persuade your dinner date to explore your naughty bits, his fumblings screened by a long tablecloth, while you spoonfeed each other this sumptuous sweet!

ASPARAGUS

Deliciously decadent when nibbled from your lover's fingers, as is corn on the cob. Drench in butter and feed each other.

STRAWBERRIES AND CREAM

Mouthwatering and can be so erotic. Feed your lover strawberries that have been dipped into a bowl of caster sugar and whipped cream. You can add to the fun by blindfolding your lover to get you both really messy and your mouths literally smothered in cream.

CHOCOLATE ECLAIR

I am a self-confessed chocaholic with a very sweet tooth. There's something very symbolic about a chocolate eclair – the way the cream simply oozes out when you first bite into it makes me adore eating one slowly and seductively in front of my man of the moment.

Those are a few of my edible favourites. A girlfriend of mine, Angie, told me her favourite erotic food is barbecued spare ribs. She then went on to tell me that she and her lover devour their favourite dish in the bath. I asked her to elaborate, and here's her recipe and her recommended modus operandi.

A STICKY MESS IN THE BATH

10 Chinese spare ribs marinated in soya sauce, red wine, pepper and salt
2 heaped dessertspoons of sugar
Chopped garlic to taste
A teaspoonful of paprika, chilli, tabasco and ginger
The juice of an orange
A splash of Grand Marnier or Cointreau
Half a cup of vinegar

In a large pan brown the meat. Add the garlic and spices. Pour in the vinegar and simmer until most of the liquid has evaporated. Add the orange, liqueur and sugar. Retain on the heat until the meat is tender and gooey in texture.

Meanwhile, run the bath and add some scented oils. Light your bathroom with candles. Climb into the bath and serve the meal in large bowls floating in the bathtub. Feast away, feeding each other with your fingertips. Use two small bowls for bones, the bath water for finger bowls and each other's bodies as napkins.

On that fingerlicking note I think it's time to get kinky!

LET'S RECAP!

- 'I once received a letter from a gentleman whose favoured fantasy was for me to munch a ring doughnut off his dick!'
- 'I've always longed for a man who would go crazy at the thought of shoving an ice-cream cornet straight up my snatch, then eating it out.'
- 'When he lowered his head to tackle the strawberry nestled between my cunt lips, I was moaning and squirming, and beside myself with excitement.'
- 'It was certainly an arousing experience having dozens of men and women feasting on my body, not to mention the fumbling fingers that delighted in smearing sticky honey all over and up my cunt.'
- 'I cut a hole in the top of the water melon, pour in a little hot water, then fuck it. I highly recommend it!'
- 'If you're not completely sure that your other half will be eager to join you in a splatterfest *extraordinaire*, do broach the subject before scrunching a black forest gâteau down the front of his or her panties!'

12

Kinky!

In the bizarre world labelled 'kinky', we encounter a new spectrum of personal taste. Some reading this book may well consider that in previous chapters, I've already delved into the murky waters of deviance, and think that depilation, fistfucking or sticking a penis into a ripe water melon is somewhat perverse behaviour. Who knows? What *is* the norm? If your lover starts expressing an interest in water sports, spanking or exhibitionism, then my advice to you would be to decide whether or not you think you could enjoy kinky sex. I think it is important that you experiment a little. You may in fact discover that something that sounds absolutely disgusting feels absolutely fabulous! But if, after trying it, it isn't your bag, you must make a stand. Perhaps you could arrive at a happy medium that keeps you both satisfied.

Personally my philosophy is that as long as an activity involves consenting adults and no other member of society is caused any harm, people should be allowed to enjoy their weird and wonderful pleasures to the full.

In 1990 there was a test case at the Old Bailey, called 'Operation Spanner', in which a group of men were found guilty of practising heavy sadomasochism on themselves and each other. For this 'depraved' behaviour the courts dished out some fairly lengthy prison sentences. This fiasco cost the country millions and in my view was a complete waste of taxpayers' money. Unfortunately, Great Britain in the late eighties and the early nineties seems to me to be a haven for vociferous spoilsports and bigots who excel in forcing their ignorant views upon others. In the European Community, where sexual liberation is tolerated in every other member state, the Brits believe that we are right and all the others are wrong! Not the vast majority of British people, but a small minority, with big mouths, the hypocritical establishment and the powers that be which are slowly but surely attempting to suppress our sexual freedom and personal choice. Remember November 1989 when the Labour MP Claire Short abandoned her campaign to ban Page Three girls, and made a vain attempt to sweep erotic magazines from high-street shops! Monstrous, eh?

I will handle the eccentricities of kinky sex alphabetically, and if I should dare to omit your idiosyncrasy, I offer my sincere apologies in advance. I suspect there are some unique sexual phenomena that even I haven't discovered yet!

BONDAGE

At the outset I would like to separate bondage from SM, although they are obviously related. Lovers of SM, rubber, spanking, and especially domination often have a keen interest in bondage. Bondage can vary to an enormous degree. I enjoy being tethered to my four-poster bed, and adore being fucked relentlessly when rendered helpless. On the other hand, I am stimulated by tying up my man and teasing him unmercifully. Both of those activities I would class as light bondage. At the other end of the scale I was talking to a middle-aged gent at a party recently who informed me that he is constantly incarcerated in a form of chastity belt which renders him unable ever to reach erection. The only time his dominant female partner removes his restraint is for daily washing. Now that I would term heavy bondage. The guy laughed as he told me his embarrassing predicament every time he passes through the metal detectors at airports!

Even heavier bondage involves being locked away in cupboards or cramped closets for hours on end, and being hung from ceilings while trussed up like turkeys. Extreme bondish fetishists get their kicks from the feelings of maschochistic helplessness. They are generally male and spend more time relishing knots, chains and manacles than dreaming of wet cunts. All sorts of restrictive gear, including straitjackets, gas masks, manacles, handcuffs and chastity belts, are available from specialist shops.

I know several couples who indulge in fairly heavy bondage. A few of them have even set aside a room in their home for bondage play. But many lovers of bondage are forced to pay for their kicks. A friend of mine, Lindi St Clair, leader of the Corrective Party and a working dominatrix, told me: 'Many of my clients are eminent businessmen and high-powered executives. Politicians, royalty and aristocracy come to me for sexual release.'

Your lover probably doesn't stretch to these bondage extremes — if so I'm sure you'd already be aware of it! Obviously all bondage etiquette requires both partners to know exactly how far to go. Mutual trust is imperative. Make sure you know your partner well before you indulge in any form of bondage, and never tie anything around the neck. There are people who get a kick out of strangulation, but sometimes one can go just a little too far in the search for erotic thrills!

EXHIBITIONISM AND VOYEURISM

I suppose you could call me an exhibitionist, a bit of a show-off in fact. I like to wind people up by behaving in a rude and almost indecent manner, and I'm a bit of a voyeur also — I get off on watching others have a good time. Exhibitionists get an extra kick from knowing that they are being observed by others, and to be at their happiest, they should team up with voyeurs. Exhibitionist females delight in wearing short skirts and no knickers in public places. And when the time is right they award complete strangers a quick flash of their hairy havens, which in turn excites their voyeuristic partner no end. Exhibitionist couples frequently invite a third party to witness, or join in with their lovemaking. 'Dogging', which I mentioned in a previous chapter, is an outlet for many voyeurs and exhibitionists.

Here's a letter that I received from a voyeur:

I guess I'm one of those lucky bums who has a randy cock-loving bitch as a wife. Hannah loves cock, any man's cock as long as it's long and thick and preferably black. She reckons a black man's skin compliments her creamy white skin to perfection. I love to watch her being fucked and then to do her with my tongue when her fella's finished. I love to lick fresh love juice from her pussy. I've loaned my wife to other men ever since we got married two months ago. Mind you, I've been doing it for several years now and she has a string of big-cocked men to service her. Of late she's been having two or three a night.

This is only one of hundred of letters I've been sent by voyeurs. I printed a letter in a similar vein in

Penthouse magazine and it seemed to open the floodgates. Voyeurs from all over the country were writing to me to tell how much sexual stimulation could be achieved from watching their partners get fucked by another. The old green-eyed monster, jealousy, just didn't enter into it.

Now here's a letter sent to me from an exhibitionist called Joy. She wrote:

John and I have been married for over ten years, but we still manage to keep the spice in our love life. That's because of my particular penchant for flashing. I'm a pure exhibitionist. If you asked me how I would spend a perfect evening, I would tell you that it would be to dress up like a complete tart, go out on the town with my husband and flash my cunt at as many unsuspecting males as I can. I'd go into my routine in quiet country pubs, posh restaurants and even at football matches. The confused yet delighted look that crosses a bloke's face when he gets an eyeful of my hairy beaver makes my juices boil.

The other night it went one step further. John and I were in a quiet country pub in the middle of nowhere. I was dressed in my usual exhibitionist garb: plenty of make-up, my lips painted glossy red, my long blonde hair piled on top, my heaving bosom peering out of the neckline of my figure-hugging dress, which was short enough to reveal stocking tops. My long legs were encased in sheer stockings and my feet in high-heeled patent court shoes. Naturally I wasn't wearing any panties. The lounge bar was almost empty. There was not a single candidate for our fun and games in sight until a young man in his early twenties came into the bar. He was quite cute looking, and dressed rather smartly in a dark suit. He appealed to me at once, so I gave John the signal and waited for the newcomer to buy a drink and sit down.

As luck would have it, he sat down only a couple of tables from us, directly facing me. I sprang into action. Firstly crossing and uncrossing my legs to attract his attention. He fixed his eyes upon me immediately, so I coyly sipped my drink and slowly spread my legs to reveal my stocking tops and my hairy fanny in all its glory. The look that crossed his face was one of pure glee and he wasted no time at all in coming over and joining us. This had never happened before and although I felt a little strange I welcomed this new dimension to my flashing game.

He asked if he could buy us a drink. We accepted, and while he was up at the bar I asked John what he thought of the situation. John asked me if I fancied the bloke, and I admitted that I did. Then my husband winked at me and said: 'Well if you want him, fuck him!'

I was still open-mouthed when he returned to our table with the drinks. I was also very wet between the thighs. He sat next to me and within moments, one of his hands had come to rest on my knee. I was trembling all over as Bill, our new-found friend, slid his hand dangerously higher and higher up my leg.

'Shall we all go outside?' I ventured, as it was a pleasantly warm evening. John and Bill said nothing, just smiled at each other, then got up and followed me from the bar.

Once in the car park John invited Bill to fuck me while he watched. Bill fell to his knees and slid his tongue into my hot hole, simultaneously fingering me as he flicked my clit with his tongue.

167

I leaned back against the bonnet of our car, let my short skirt ride up, arched my back, and thrust my cunt into his face. I could hear shouts of encouragement from my husband as he stood right next to us. His cock was in his hand; he wanked it faster and faster. I squealed as I came twice in a matter of minutes.

'Fuck her, why don't you!' implored John, so Bill swiftly got up, grabbed me by the hips and turned me around. I heard him unzip his fly, and the very next minute his throbbing cock was slipping oh-so-delightfully into my snatch as I bent over the bonnet of the car. He fucked me using long, deliberate strokes, his thick cock filling me to the hilt. His speed picked up and I heard him muttering that he was about to spunk. I could hear John building to orgasm as well.

Soon after, I felt two lots of hot come; one spurting forcefully up inside me, the other splattering over my arse cheeks as my husband and a complete stranger released their cream together.

A mate of mine, Mike, told me his voyeuristic tale.

I was in Los Angeles on business and I'd met this very attractive girl. We were up in her hotel room and I was getting pretty serious with my head between her legs when a key turned in the door and this bloke walked in. I stopped immediately, assuming that there was going to be some kind of row, but to my surprise this bloke stuck out his hand and introduced himself. Then his girlfriend pushed me back between her legs, and I carried on where I'd left off. All the while, her boyfriend stood watching us. I even fucked her with her boyfriend sitting down carefully observing us. He wasn't wanking, just watching intently.

INFANTILISM

There are grown men and women who get off on being dressed in a nappy, sucking on a dummy and spending a lot of time sitting in a playpen listening to kiddies' stories. 'Spanking and nappy training are both an integral part of the sexual thrill for adult babies,' I was told by a keen enthusiast. He went on to reveal more about his particular kink: 'If a man or woman shows interest in regression to childhood, this should be encouraged as it will help them to relax and ease their tension. It should however be done properly, and in such a way to give pleasure to both the male and female. Take some trouble over the dressing up, and select an age for the baby. Usually the age of around three or four is about right. What provides the excitement is the dressing-up, the being cuddled, sucking a dummy or a bottle, the nappy training, spanking and the baby talk. This will all stimulate the adult baby into masturbation.'

Each year at the Sex Maniacs' Ball there is a playpen at the disposal of people who get a thrill from behaving as an adult baby, although my source did tell me: 'The very suggestion that someone other than the adult baby's partner is going to be allowed to see them in this condition sends unpleasant shivers down the spine.' Obviously some adult babies are happy to 'come out', and others aren't.

LEATHER AND RUBBER

Wearing leather and rubber offers a second skin, a feeling of power, and a recognised identity. Often there is a fetishist effect that makes the wearer or their partner instantly orgasmic. Some can climax from merely polishing and buffing their rubber attire. Rubber in particular has some peculiar sensual qualities. It has a distinctive smell, it clings, and it makes you sweat a lot. Rubber and leather fanatics have their own magazines, their own clubs, and shops that cater just for their specific taste.

SADOMASOCHISM

Some people confuse sexual rituals between consenting adults with violent abusive behaviour. What they fail to understand is that in SM the understanding between the two people is far more significant than the whip or cane. There is a little touch of the sadist in us all, and on the whole, people who use SM in their sex play work out their dominant/submissive feelings and behave like ordinary human beings in their everyday life.

One reason SM is so popular is that for some people, pain and pleasure seem to be interchangeable. Certainly the pain and pleasure areas of the brain are very close. When you get very excited it becomes simple for those feelings to intermingle. Intense pain can be felt as intense pleasure. There are people who agree to live their lives on a full-time basis of domination and submission. The sub often has as much control as the dom in this kind of relationship because they demand or beg for certain punishment and conditions. Subs are just as likely to be male as female, and the same goes for doms. There are far more subs crying out to be dominated than there are doms, which makes a nonsense of the accusation that SM is all about female degradation.

There is a certain etiquette that doms should follow while out in SM clubs:

- Find out if whipping is allowed and how heavy it can be.
- Never whip anyone without their permission.
- Don't ask someone else's slave to perform a task for you without first asking their master or mistress.

Spanking, flagellation, and smothering your partner's naked body with hot candle wax are just some of the games played during SM love play. Body piercing is also very popular, as SM fans enjoy wearing decorative body jewellery on their nipples, labia, foreskin and so on. Do make sure you know and trust your partner before participating in anything of this kind. I have limited personal experience of SM, although I have many friends who are lovers of this sexual genre. I have on several occasions attended SM clubs where impromptu beatings and spankings take place.

Around ten years ago I met up with photographer/filmmaker George Harrison-Marks who asked me if I wanted to take part in some of his productions. Always eager to learn, I appeared in one of his films as a traffic warden that got a good spanking. I could hardly sit down for a week! Then I reversed roles, and in another movie I played the part of a dominatrix called Madame Monique who spanked, whipped and caned just about everybody who came near her! Actually the film is still available in Europe if by chance you should like to view a copy of my early dom performance!

I quite enjoyed dressing up as the traffic warden and having my bottom slapped by a handsome, young London cabbie. I found the warm glow of a smarting bottom quite arousing. During sex, if I'm on top straddling my partner, I enjoy a firm hand slapping my bottom just as I'm beginning to climax. But as the aggressive Madame Monique, I didn't enjoy the domination. I loved dressing up in sexy, tight leather gear and shouting orders at everybody, but when it actually came down to whacking — well, I didn't like it one bit. I did learn, however, that there is a right way and wrong way to do it. All of the people I had to cane or whip were well into it, and explained that it is important to know where and when to whip, and that an enormous amount of mutual trust is involved, especially if the sub is restrained in any way.

I remember flippantly writing in a magazine article once, 'I love a man who knows how to beg'. I was inundated with offers from willing slaves promising their absolute devotion, but I declined their kind offers!

TRANSVESTISM

There is a very famous model called Tula, or Caroline Cossey, who started out life as a boy called Barry (although she says, 'I was born a girl with male genitalia'), had a sex change in her late teens and became a fabulous-looking woman. When I first started my modelling career, I recall turning up at various castings and bumping into Tula. More often than not Tula would get the modelling job, because as a glamour model she was the tops, appearing in massive advertising campaigns and even as a Bond girl. Tula is in fact a transexual. Thousands of sex-change operations take place each year and produce beautiful new women. Many decide to have silicone implants to give them breasts. Or, alternatively, hormones will do the trick. A brand-new pussy is created for them during surgery, but some opt to keep their dicks, and can still achieve erection. I've seen some interesting European movies where the transexual has both!

I have an American friend called Shannon, a stunningly attractive woman in her early thirties who was born a man. She became a top American porno star in transvestite movies, appearing as a woman, complete with silicone breasts, but retaining a dick. She moved to Germany to work as a make-up artist and finally had the full operation, fell in love and is now married to a man. She's a great girl (I've only known her as a girl, so it's difficult for me to imagine her any other way), completely outrageous and a real flirt, and she told me something that I found very interesting. While she lived as a boy she had sex only with girls. As soon as she had the final operation, she switched to men.

Some TVs prefer to live most of their life as a man and just cross-dress, using bras equipped with false cleavages, and false bottoms to create the image of hips. They learn how to use make-up and wigs, and sometimes they are assisted and advised on feminine attire and cosmetics by their wives. Some even go as far as sharing clothes with their spouses, if their wives can adjust to the situation. The ultimate thrill of the transvestite is to become somebody else, adopt a new identity, and to fool other people into believing they are a member of the opposite sex. Dressing up and adopting a temporary new gender is what stimulates and excites them. It really is as simple as that. Female-to-male transvestism is less common and less talked about. Women TVs can, with the help of hormones, grow a beard, and can have an artificial penis.

WATERSPORTS

I'm not referring to scuba-diving or seaside frolics here: no, I'm talking urolagnia, enemas and copraphagia. Let's start off with the more popular golden showers. Lots of women feel an urge to pee when they're making love. Some even find they can't stop themselves. Sexual intercourse can put pressure on the bladder and often the muscular spasms of your orgasm can make you spurt a little. Others go a little further and derive pleasure from watching each other pee on each other.

Others go even further and drink piss, shit on each other and administer enemas. If your partner requests you do it, it is obviously for you to decide whether or not you would feel happy introducing these unusual activities into your sex life. Steer well clear of anything you find degrading or humiliating; it's probably best to avoid the kind of sexual activity that makes you feel afterwards that you wish you hadn't indulged!

Kinky sex is often very individual, and some very weird and wonderful fantasies can be termed kinky. For instance, a girlfriend of mine works for a telephone sex compnay and often talks directly to the callers. One caller told her how he fantasised about being punished for drug smuggling. What excited him was the idea of being paraded through the customs hall at Heathrow airport, stark naked, with his bollocks clamped in a vice and pulled backwards between his legs. Ouch! I wonder how he thought up that one? But personalised kinks are quite common.

In addition to all the kinkiness included in this chapter, some men and women are turned on only by a particular type. There are women who choose to make love only to bald men, black men, or men with beards; some men are turned on by mature ladies, fat ladies and pregnant ladies spouting milk. And we should never forget fetishism − the ability to get off on an object or a particular part of the body.

I used to have a foot fetishist who regularly telephoned me at my London flat. More than a decade ago, my brother opened a pub in Wiltshire, and as I was a Page Three girl at the time, we decided to try for some publicity by inviting a local photographer along to the grand opening. I posed for the photographs sitting on the bartop, while my brother stood next to me. I was wearing open-toed sandals and my feet were quite prominent in the photograph that eventually turned up in one of the Sunday Nationals.

After spotting my tantalising tootsies in the newspaper, the foot fetishist tracked down my telephone number and the calls started flooding in. I don't suppose he would have continued for long if he wasn't getting satisfied. But he was getting exactly what he was after, because every time he called, my crazy flatmate, Marie Harper, would get on the extension and start exciting him by talking about sweaty toes, hard skin and how she adored licking my feet! The caller was well away, and Marie and I thought it fun. It really does take all sorts when it comes to kinks!

LET'S RECAP!

- 'Some reading this book may well consider that already I've delved into the murky waters of deviance, and think that depilation, fist-fucking or sticking a penis into a ripe water melon is somewhat perverse behaviour.'
- 'Extreme bondage fetishists get their kicks from the feelings of masochistic helplessness. They are generally male and spend more time relishing knots, chains and manacles than dreaming of wet cunts.'
- 'Hannah loves cock, any man's cock as long as it's long and thick and preferably black.'
- 'Bill fell to his knees and slid his tongue into my hot hole, simultaneously fingering me as he flicked my clit with his tongue.'
- 'During sex, if I'm on top straddling my partner, I enjoy a firm hand slapping my bottom just as I'm beginning to climax.'
- 'Lots of women feel an urge to pee when they're making love.'

13

Lezbefriends

Women who swing both ways are the subject of fascination for many men and the object of suspicion for lots of women. In this chapter I intend to delve deep into the sensual world of the bisexual woman. I have chosen to concentrate on female bisexuality because it interests and excites me a great deal, and because it is undoubtedly a favourite fantasy for many men. The idea of watching two beautiful women romantically pleasing each other with trembling fingers and flickering tongues, heightened by the supposition that they may in time turn their attention to the horny voyeur, is one that turns grown men into dribbling, drooling wrecks!

Although a common fantasy for males, we women are far less likely to have erotic fantasies involving two men screwing each other, though porno star Paula Price told me how she fantasised about seeing her boyfriend being fucked by another man, and an ex-colleague of mine from *Penthouse* magazine revealed to me how she longed to fulfil her most forbidden fantasy – peeping through a blind to ogle two hairy, virile men shafting each other vigorously. It is not, however, a typical female fantasy. In fact, the very idea of men making love to each other can be a complete turn-off to both men and women alike.

Bisexuals are an emerging group, coming out in the way the gay community has done for the past twenty years. Probably about a third of the population is bisexual, but many of this number are unaware of their bisexuality.

To be bisexual is to have the potential to be open emotionally and sexually to people as people, regardless of their gender. This usually leads to a unique approach to sex. Bisexuals usually make great lovers and are frequently very highly sexed. Bi women and men can find themselves in pure lesbian or homosexual relationships, then, when that relationship has run its course, they may well find that their next involvement is completely heterosexual. One could assume that finding a suitable partner is much easier for bisexuals because they have twice as many lovers to choose from, but things aren't quite as simple as that! Some bisexuals feel that they might never meet any one person who could fulfil all their sexual and emotional needs.

Setting aside bisexuals for a moment, let us consider the confirmed lesbian. They seem to me to be a different breed altogether. Many lesbians sever relationships with males because of physical or mental abuse from previous male partners. After such a bad experience they want nothing more to do with men and turn to the softness of another woman for comfort and solace. Being in the business of standing up for sexual freedom in a country that so frequently wants to repress us, I often come across lesbian types who have a keen dislike of the opposite sex. Probably because of some previous bad experience, their main goal in life is to stop men enjoying their sexuality. This is not always the case, though. There is an organisation, Feminists Against Censorship, made up mainly of gay women who campaign enthusiastically for sexual freedom for homosexual and heterosexuals alike.

Although I have male friends who are bisexual, and also many gay male friends, they seem to me more private in regard to their sex lives, whereas the bisexual females I know and love enjoy nothing better than spilling the beans about their loving in graphic detail. Their very first sexual awakening with a member of their own sex is generally stimulating and enlightening, the taboo of lesbianism making it all the more erotic. Here's a letter I received from Tina who tells me of her illicit bisexual love affair:

I've been happily married for six years. I'm twenty-six years old, reasonably attractive and a bit of a nymphomaniac. Since I've been with my husband, I've always found the need to fuck other men. That doesn't mean I think any the less of him. None of my sexual activities could be classed as a real affair. I used to meet one guy in the woods regularly for a nice outdoor fuck. Another guy used to shag me in the front of his classic sports car, and from time to time, I've played around with my boss.

Anyway, that was all in the past, I've now met somebody who I seem to have a kind of obsession with, and it's a she! Sometimes I just can't concentrate on anything else. All the time I am dreaming about having sex with this beautiful woman. Until recently I'd never even thought about having sex with a woman. I've always been the kind of girl who likes to feel a nice stiff dick between my legs. What started me off was one evening when my husband was out working and I was reading an erotic magazine that featured photographs of two stunning models together. All of a sudden I could feel my cunt go all twitchy, so I slid my fingers inside my knickers and started to finger my clit to orgasm.

After that night I started to dream about making it with another woman, but I had no idea where I would find a tasty cunt to play around with. That is, until the new couple John and Sheila moved in across the road. Now John is the kind of guy I'd usually be desperate to get inside me, but not this time. Oh no, it was Sheila that I wanted. She had just turned twenty-two and was a real stunner: long dark hair, big eyes, a great figure with lovely big tits and a rounded arse. I wanted so much to strip her naked and lick her body from top to bottom. So I made it my goal to seduce her.

It was a piece of cake! Being neighbours I started inviting her over on Saturdays for a coffee. One particular Saturday afternoon, when the two men had gone to football, I invited her over for a natter. Well, that's what I told her anyway! We sat next to each other on the sofa and as the film on TV was very old, I asked if she'd like to watch a video. She agreed and so I put on the dirtiest lesbian video I could find.

On screen, two very pretty girls started to kiss each other. I glanced at Sheila. She was squirming a little. Her eyes were wide as I reached over and placed my hand on her knee. She pushed her crotch forward and sighed as my hand travelled up beneath her skirt to stroke her inner thighs. She was wearing tight white panties, and I started to rub her through her knickers. Very quickly I found her clit and massaged it with my thumb while hooking my other fingers inside her pants, sliding them into her juicy pussy. By now she had slumped down on the sofa and was thrusting her pelvis like crazy as I fingered her to a very quick orgasm.

After her first climax we started all over again, but this time much more slowly. Without rushing, we stripped each other naked, caressing and touching each other's bodies, both exploring the full delights of another woman's body for the very first time. I lay on top of Sheila and ran my hands all over her beautiful body. I kissed and sucked her fabulous breasts and then buried my face into her hairy pussy. I've never tasted a female's juices before, and Sheila's cunt tasted divine.

Together we manoeuvred ourselves into the sixty-nine position. I spread her pussy like a delicate flower and explored her with my tongue. I could feel her gentle fingers pushing inside me as her tongue slid up and down my slit. I was shivering with excitement as I eased my thumb into her arse while still licking her open pussy furiously. The sucking and fingering was all too much and seconds later we were clinging together, shouting and squealing as we orgasmed together.

That first time was simply electric. Now we meet up every Saturday afternoon and one evening in the week as well. We haven't told our husbands. It's our little secret. But somehow, I think if they found out they would be quite turned on by the thought of their wives sucking and slurping each other's pussies!

Tina is obviously the best one to judge the situation, but I would say she's probably correct in her assumption that her husband would be more turned on than upset if he found out about her 'affair'. I know of many women who have carried on affairs of this nature for years. Their regular partners or husbands know all about it and don't seem to mind, possibly because they don't see it as a real threat, more as a sexy game that their lover plays. And of course they might just want to be involved and make this happy twosome an ecstatic threesome. A photographer friend of mine has just gone to work in the States for six weeks, and I asked him what his girlfriend Laura thought of him leaving her alone for so long. He chuckled as he replied that Laura had told him she intended to find herself a pretty young girl to keep her amused. He didn't seem to mind one bit, but I suspect he would if she'd told him she was going to find herself a young male lover to while away the winter nights!

Personally I've never had a serious lesbian relationship, although on many occasions I have enjoyed playing around with bisexual women, and sometimes, when men get on my nerves, I swear I'm going to find myself a good woman to settle down with! I do find women's bodies arousing, especially as many of my girlfriends and acquaintances are models and so have stunningly attractive figures anyway. When I masturbate, one thing guaranteed to bring me off almost immediately is the memory of lesbian experiences I have had. In addition to this fantasising, I only have to think of the foxy females that I know who absolutely adore the taste of pussy, and imagine them giving my cunt a good tongue-bath, whilst my fumbling fingers are frigging away between my legs. And bingo, I'm coming in no time. My feelings are exactly the same with erotic magazines or films, my preference being for the explicit lesbian loving photographs and imagery. Call me an old romantic, call me a raving dyke, call me a wanker — I just don't care!

There seems to be a general consensus of opinion that women eat pussy differently to the way men do.

I suppose it is because some men can be a little rough, whereas all women know how delicate and sensitive a pussy is, and treat it accordingly. I've never yet had a girl lick my pussy too roughly, but I've had plenty of fellas that I've had to teach to handle my precious little puss properly! I asked a few women to tell me their views and techniques on the subject.

Julia, a twenty-eight-year-old stripper, said: 'Women are so much better at oral sex. There are two different ways to come in my opinion, oral stimulation and fucking. Men are just for fucking!'

I asked bisexual porn star Madison whom she considered eats pussy the best, men or women: 'Well, if you're going to generalise, the answer would be girls. But you do have a few guys out there who went to the school of pussy eating that were taught by girls and now are real good!'

Jane, a twenty-seven-year-old model from Kent, told me: 'I love having my pussy eaten – well, don't we all, darling? Women are different, but not better than men. When I go down on a girl, I like to watch a dildo or vibrator sliding in and out of her pussy. And I always hope she likes anal, so I can play with her arse – stick a vibrator up it while I open her pussy and very slowly lick her clit, using lots of saliva and very slow, long movements of the tongue. That's the way I like to be licked.'

Sex toys play a very important role for bisexuals, as bisexual women frequently yearn for that dick substitute to achieve full satisfaction. Double-ended dildoes are great fun for a hot, dirty lesbian session. I first spotted them in an American porn film and have been a fan of them ever since. They are generally made of pliable latex, are available in all sorts of garish colours, and are often bloody enormous! Two huge dildos are joined together at the base end, enabling horny lesbos to feel a large, soft, pricklike member filling their hot pulsating pussies to the brim. And the position that the two women have to adopt to be simultaneously fucked by the double-ended dildo makes sure that their thrusting pussies are bang on to each other for added friction and fun.

When playing around with double dildoes, it's a good idea to get hold of your rubber dicky and stay with it. Don't in the heat of the moment swap ends! For safe sex purposes it is always advisable to keep to your own sex toys and make sure you wash them after every steamy session. Other lesbian sexual practices that adhere to the rules of safe sex are kissing on the lips, the breasts and all over the body, including the pussy, as long as you have no cuts in your mouth. The same applies to fingering — cuts on the hands and fingers could be risky.

Role-playing often plays a part in many bisexual relationships — the dominant lesbian and the submissive one are a common couple. This is sometimes because one half of the partnership is experienced in lesbian loving, and the other often a total newcomer. But this is not always the case; many sexy scenes between women involve a 'boss' just because that's the way the girls get an additional thrill.

Adult movie star Porsche Lynn told me her views on role-playing: 'I'm very bisexual and I'm used to going out picking up women and bringing them home. Sometimes with girls I'm dominant, but often that's just because of my body size — I'm 5'8" and weigh 125 lbs. I'm very turned on by black women and exotic women. Actually I picked up a girl a couple of nights ago at a magic club. The next day I took her shopping and bought her some sexy lingeries, a pair of nipple clamps and a couple of whips. Then we went home and I had her try on all these outfits and we played around

184

for the rest of the day with all the new toys. We had a ball!'

Porsche seems happy to make the first move, but that can be quite a problem for some women who fancy a dalliance with another female. Where the hell do you find such a sexy creature? And when you find a woman that you fancy, how do you know if that feeling is reciprocated? Chatting up a woman for the specific purpose of lesbian sex could potentially be the most embarrassing moment of a woman's life if she's read the situation incorrectly. I don't think the Lesbian and Gay Centre in London is probably the best venue either! The way I've always ended up in a lesbian situation is by slowly getting to know another female, reading and judging a sexual undercurrent. Mind you, I'm quite lucky in that regard, because lots of the women I know are game for anything! There are, however, swing-type clubs and activities going on around the country, and perhaps you might be able to find what you're looking for at one of these social gatherings.

That very first lesbian encounter is a subject that interests me a great deal. A friend of mine, Nicki, a twenty-six-year-old stockbroker, told me a very sexy story of her first bisexual awakening which resulted from a pick-up in the back of a London cab!

One day last week I'd had a very hectic working day, but I agreed to meet a couple of colleagues in a wine bar in the West End. I couldn't face the tube, so I hailed a cab. Just as I was climbing into the black taxi, the other door opened and I came face to face with this stunning-looking woman. I remember mentally admiring her Nordic good looks before thinking, what's this woman doing in my cab? She smiled at me, and asked where I was heading. I told her Oxford Street, and as she was heading in the same direction we agreed to share the taxi.

The trip from the City to the West End in rush hour took a while. She told me her name was Cheryl and she worked as a travel executive. I was sitting opposite her on the long bench seat, while she was seated on one of the pull-down chairs. Every few minutes she crossed her long, slender legs and rewarded me with a flash of black stocking tops. I couldn't for the life of me understand why I was so attentive, but I could feel my eyes drawn to her hemline, hoping that her navy pinstripe skirt would ride up just a little higher to give me a glimpse of her panties. I was fascinated by her manicured hands that she used expansively when she talked. She brushed them against her pouty lips, stroked her throat with her fingers and seemed to be tracing a line from her neck down to her breasts. I was mesmerised by her, and for some completely alien reason, I wanted her to be as interested in me as I was in her.

I could feel a dampness seeping into my knickers as I leaned back in my seat and opened my legs a little. She spotted it at once and for a full ten seconds or so stared hard at my parted knees. Then, slowly she leant towards me, placed a hand on my knee and asked me if my appointment could wait. Afraid to answer, I just nodded my head, and with that she sat alongside me.

Her hand kept constant contact with me, but began to climb. The sensation of her talonlike fingernails snaking up my leg made me quiver. With her face close to mine, looking me right in the eyes, she told me in a slow even voice that she was going to take me home and eat out my sweet little pussy. My heart was pounding as I told her that I would like that. By now I could actually feel my cunt twitching. Her fingertips crept around to the inside of my thigh and continued to travel upwards. She leant forwards and kissed me, and as her tongue probed my mouth, her fingers made first contact with my pussy. I started to come immediately, even before she pulled my knickers off to one side and gently caressed my swollen cunt lips. As her fingers gently opened me up, I was still coming. My whole body started to spasm as she found my clitoris and tenderly stroked it. Two or three fingers slipped inside me and I was still coming.

Transfixed in a sort of a sexual trance, I felt the cab come to a halt. My eyes flickered open to see Cheryl sucking her fingers and smiling mischieviously at me. She pulled down my skirt, paid the driver and helped me out. On the way up to her apartment I explained that I'd never been with a woman before. Cheryl giggled naughtily and told me that she knew that, and assured me that I would love it. She was right.

Once inside she undressed me incredibly slowly. One by one she slipped the buttons on my shirt, caressing my bare shoulders as she removed it. Nibbling my earlobes and kissing my neck, she gingerly squeezed my breasts, her forefingers flicking my nipples through the lace of my bra. Prior to this, I was standing, but at this moment I sank to my knees. Cheryl unclasped my bra and let my breasts swing free. My nipples were so hard they were almost painful as she drew them one by one into her mouth, gripping each nipple with her teeth. Kneeling together on the floor of her lounge, she thrust her knee between my splayed thighs and nuzzled it firmly against my cunt. As she gorged on my tits, I rubbed my hot cunt against her stockinged knee.

It all got a bit wild then as we both tore at each other's clothes, desperate to abandon all that was inhibiting us from exploring each other's excited bodies. I distinctly recall seeing Cheryl's breasts for the first time. She had pert breasts with pink nipples that pointed skywards. A perfect mouthful is how I would describe them. Saliva dripped from my mouth as I ran my tongue all over them. All the while I feasted on them, Cheryl finger-fucked me, sliding two fingers in and out of my juicy cunt.

Particularly sweet was when Cheryl bent me over the sofa so my bottom was hoisted high in the air. Her long fingernails tantalisingly fondling my buttocks, creeping nearer and nearer to my creamy crack until finally one warm hand reached through and grabbed handfuls of my hairy cunt before zeroing in and fingering my clit. She used her other hand to open up my cunt lips, smoothing away my thick thatch of dark hair, making plenty of room for that slippery, soft tongue of hers. By this time I'd lost count of the number of times I'd come, and I'd not yet tasted her cunt!

It was in her bedroom that I first got to sample her sweet nectar. Still dressed in a navy garter belt and stockings, she made herself comfortable on her king-size bed and, with one hand pulling back the tip of her slit, in a breathy voice she invited me to taste her. A little nervous at first, I lay between her knees and came face to face with her glorious golden pussy. Unlike mine, it was covered with feathery, silken blonde hair and was very neatly trimmed. Her lips were bulging and her cunt simply dripped with sexual juices. I lowered my face to it and breathed in her heady aroma. Grabbing me by my hair she raised my head and groaned that she would teach me to eat pussy. But, she told me to wait and watch while she fingered herself, so that I could see exactly what she liked. I stared at this beautiful blonde cunt while her flashing red fingernails went to work. As her fingers pumped in and out, I couldn't resist sliding my tongue onto her clit. Her fingers and my tongue were a blur as she peaked, clawing at my hair, calling out my name as she thrashed around in ecstasy.

Naughty Nicki! I enjoyed her story so much that I interviewed another first-timer. Her name is Gina and she's a twenty-one-year-old secretary.

Linzi: *Do you enjoy sex with men and women?*

Gina: Yes, I lost my virginity to a man when I was sixteen years old. It was fun. I like sex with men, but I've always had a longing to try it with a woman.

Linzi: *Tell me about your first time with a woman.*

Gina: A bit of a long story, but here goes. In my office at work, I have a lady boss. She's very competent, in her early thirties and very attractive. She seemed to take to me and sometimes after work we'd go out for a meal together. We got to the stage that I'd often drop round to her flat for a coffee and a gossip.

Well, one night I had a really bad row with this guy I was seeing and was very upset. On the off-chance that my boss would be in, I called on her. She was lovely, gave me a stiff drink, comforted me and basically let me cry on her shoulder. But as we sat together embracing on

189

the sofa, the atmosphere somehow seemed to change. Subtly, smoothly, but unmistakably. Instinctively I knew where it might lead if I gave the right signals. So I did just that, by eye contact and by moving my body as she touched me.

It was quite different from making love to a man. We just stroked each other very softly, our lips meeting in a warm, tender kiss. We undressed each other so slowly, and then she pulled me close. I felt our breasts crush together, and her long, freshly washed hair brush across my face. For a long time we just lay together enjoying the embrace, letting our thighs mingle, kissing and caressing. She gently rolled me on to my back and began to move her fingers all over my body. At each stroke her light touch moved lower and lower, until I could hardly wait for her fingertips to touch me there! I felt my thighs opening in anticipation, and when I thought, this is it, she started running her fingertips along my inner thighs. No man had ever made me wait that long, and by the time I felt her fingers brush against my pussy, I was ecstatic!

She did exactly what I wanted, finding my clitoris instantly and fingering me with great finesse. I wanted to do the same to her, so I plunged my hand between her legs and she felt wonderful.

Linzi: *Did she use her tongue on you?*

Gina: Did she ever! It was so different. She gently opened my lips wide with her fingertips and very lightly teased my slit. Then she started to rub her nose all over my pussy, breathing me in, enjoying my sexual smell. Her soft hair sort of

190

tickled the inside of my thighs as she started to lick me faster and a little harder. I was clinging on to her hair, moaning and crying out as she feasted on me before inserting a manicured fingernail inside my wet, wet pussy, which just made me cream and cream!

Linzi: *Was that first time with your boss the first of many sexual experiences with women?*

Gina: Yes, I still fuck guys, but at the moment I favour lesbian sex. Actually the next thing I want to try is having a two-girl, one-guy threesome!

Nicki and Gina both seem to concur that a lesbian lovemaking session involves a slow sensuous build-up which, along with the taboo element, affords the lesbo lovers one hell of a time! It's convenient that Gina should conclude as she did, because now we move swiftly along to a chapter that explores the world of troilism, orgies, group sex — in fact, the more the merrier!

LET'S RECAP!

- 'The concept of watching two beautiful women romantically pleasing each other with trembling fingers and flickering tongues, heightened by the supposition that they may in time turn their attention on the horny voyeur, is one that turns grown men into dribbling, drooling wrecks!'

- 'Sometimes when men get on my nerves, I swear I'm going to find myself a good woman to settle down with!'

- 'When I masturbate, one thing that is guaranteed to bring me off almost immediately is to bring to mind lesbian experiences that I've had in my life.'

- 'There are two different ways to come in my opinion; oral stimulation and there's fucking. Men are just for fucking!'

- 'When I go down on a girl, I like to watch a dildo or vibrator sliding in and out of her pussy. And I always hope she likes anal, so I can play with her arse.'

- 'She used her other hand to open my cunt lips, smoothing away my thick thatch of dark hair, making plenty of room for that slippery, soft tongue of hers.'

14

The More the Merrier!

Could you bear the idea of sharing your lover? What would be your reaction, girls, if your partner suggested that another man and woman join you and your lover in bed? Or how would you react, guys, if your partner wanted another woman to join you for sex? Swinging, swapping, orgies and threesomes are a great topic for discussion. Are they the perfect way to spice up your sex life, or are they more likely to end in disaster? Naturally that depends on the individuals involved in the swinging sex. If you and your partner think you can handle it, stick to the important rules of safe sex, and try it!

There are many honest ways of enjoying safe sex with more than one partner. You can be single and have several relationships. You can have an open marriage and enjoy sex with other partners, or you can even live in a group relationship, known as polyfidelity. But by far the most popular swinging activity these days (aside from troilism, which we'll get to later) is swapping, a recreation where couples meet up specifically for sex. Swapping sprang up in the sixties and continues to be practised and enjoyed today, whether the sex takes place in private homes, swing clubs or impromptu orgies. It can be a practical way to remain in a stable relationship whilst still enjoying variety in your sex life.

..r, swapping works only if you operate as a ..ple and you both desire the freedom. If one partner is reluctant and is coerced into swapping, it will all undoubtedly end in tears!

When a couple decide to meet up with another couple to have sex, one partner in each relationship often plays a dominant role – probably the person who came up with the idea in the first place! If your lover suggests you indulge in swinging or swapping, and you feel that you don't want to get involved or can't handle the situation, don't feel obliged. The decision is yours! Perhaps you should consider whether or not you're being creative enough in your sex life? Remember, swapping isn't the swift answer to all sex problems. However, many swingers feel that swapping partners brings them closer together. Once you've seen your husband or wife screwing another person, you have shared that emotion and there is no need to keep secrets any more.

Although clubs and contact magazines might be the easiest way to meet up with new swingers, the best parties are private, with people who come together through personal introductions. Impromptu orgies can be a celebration of sex, whilst organised orgies can be wild or a complete turn-off. Before attending this kind of event you have to come to terms with the fact that there may be unappealing people there who want sex with you, or, to put it more bluntly, partners that you wouldn't touch with a barge pole! Can you switch off, lose yourself and fuck for a fuck's sake? Can you look beneath the surface and look for inner beauty? Personally that all seems to me rather a lot to deal with when you just fancy a spontaneous fuck! And girls, if you do take part in an orgy, I think it's important not to regard it as a typical male fantasy. It has all the right ingredients to be a great female fantasy, especially if you take on two men.

194

Sensitive people don't really need to be told how to behave at swinging scenarios, but once you've arrived and nerves and excitement takes over, common sense can go out the window! The big rule is that no always means no, and you must learn to recognise jealousy.

The swing scene varies enormously, be it at a private house or at a recognised swing club. Some couples may just want to relax with like-minded people, lounge around, have a few drinks and talk explicitly about their fantasies. Others go one stage further, indulging in mutual masturbation with couples or individuals, while the more adventurous swingers move on to full-scale fucking and sucking with one or several new partners!

The most outrageous swingers of all are to be found at gang-bang parties, where an insatiable woman agrees to take on a great number of men manually, orally or whatever! I remember being at a party like this, which was organised by a girlfriend of mine, last year. The party catered for a liberated crowd, varying from heavy SM fans to voyeurs to sexy models. Halfway through the evening it was announced that a girl was about to perform. About thirty men queued up across the dance floor to be serviced by a stunning blonde dressed only in a leather bodice. She went down on her knees and sucked and wanked every one of them off, one by one. It had to be seen to be believed! And to top that, a friend of mine who works as a staff photographer for *Private*, a sexually explicit Swedish magazine, was sent to Amsterdam to photograph a reportage on a Dutch woman who was trying to beat the world record for fucking. A proper sex bed, complete with stirrups, was created, and she lay back and took on one hundred and fifty cocks in less than six hours! I've never seen so many condoms filled up with come as in this spunky magazine feature!

195

I've been to a couple of organised orgies that were choc-a-bloc with unfanciable men desperate to get laid. I beat a hasty retreat on both occasions. I did, however, attend a wondrous impromptu orgy that was held in a sex therapist's house in Earls Court. I distinctly remember a nurse called Julia who fucked about fifteen men. The party was being held in the large basement flat and Julie kept disappearing in this open-fronted Victorian lift with various men. The lift would ascend with Julia disappearing from view, hurriedly unzipping her new partner's pants. By the time the lift returned to the basement again, her partner was grinning from ear to ear and hurriedly tucking his dick away! Julia eventually tired of that little game and settled for fucking and sucking men in the centre of the room where most of the party revellers, including her husband, looked on in delight.

It was at this same party that I first sampled troilism. I had gone to the sexy social gathering in the company of a new boyfriend. Watching the frantic sexual activity all around made me and my man horny, aided by the fact that I was somewhat underdressed in an incredibly short, red skin-tight dress that flashed my bare pussy at frequent intervals. As we were both feeling hot to trot, we snuck off to an empty spare bed that was built up over the study area. We climbed up the stepladder, tucked ourselves away in this secret little corner and began to explore each other's bodies. I can't quite recall exactly how far we'd progressed when I realised all of a sudden that the fingers probing my pussy possessed talonlike fingernails! I opened my eyes and glanced towards the stepladder to see a beautiful young woman stroking and fingering my pussy! And very nice it was too.

Threesomes, on the whole, do tend to be unplanned events. Sometimes a *menage à trois* develops with two

196

females and one man because the female partner initiates the act to discover what lesbian sex is like. Women are often attracted to other women's bodies and may just want to try it once. The male invariably agrees to go along with it, as bedding his lover and another female at one time is a typical male fantasy and offers a challenge to the male ego.

I spoke to three women who had the desire to introduce a woman into their marital bed.

Laura, a married woman in her thirties, told me: 'I have a very stable relationship with my husband and we both enjoy sex to the full. We spend a lot of time discussing our fantasies. I like to be very open about sex, and told my husband Derek that I would like to bring another woman into our sex life. I even had the woman in mind, a bisexual friend of mine. We invited her round for dinner and the inevitable happened — the three of us ended up in bed. I learnt for the first time how to touch another woman, and I enjoyed stroking her breasts and licking her pussy. I came like crazy sitting on her face while my husband fucked her. It only happened that one time, but it was a wonderful sexual awakening for my husband and me.'

Beverley, a thirty-one-year-old ex-model, told me: 'I wanted to have a threesome with another woman and my boyfriend. I chose the girl and he was happy to go along with it. It was all going along great, I was getting off on letting her lick me, watching her suck my boyfriend's prick and everything, but the thing I couldn't cope with was when he was about to fuck her. I just watched his prick penetrate her for the first time and I just shouted out "no" at the top of my voice. I just couldn't bear it!'

Beautiful American sex star Savannah revealed details of her threesome fun with her rockstar boyfriend. 'He's into group sex, so when I went to his

Laguna Beach concert, I picked up this really good-looking chick. When he came off stage and saw me with her, he asked me who she was. Then I just started kissing her and playing with her, and he couldn't wait to get us back to his suite. We had a wild ol' time!'

Although sessions with two women and one man are every man's favourite fantasy, they are not always as fulfilling an encounter as when the players in this triangle of sex are two men and a girl. Threesomes involving two women can finish up with the two females making love to each other while the man droops disappointedly! When there is just one woman involved, one man can rest, watch and restore his energy while the other man keeps up the hard sex action. And if they're both ready for action at the same time, there's always her eager mouth to be filled. In a previous chapter I've touched upon voyeurism, a kind of erotic peepshow where guys get off on watching their women get fucked by another man. It is far less commonplace for women to get off on watching their man fuck another woman!

I talked to a couple of women who have taken on two men at once, not in a premeditated situation, but because they were feeling horny, and the three-way sex just happened.

Porno star and distant cousin of Dolly Parton, Julia Parton, told me her experience with two men: 'The weirdest thing I've ever done is when I slept with two brothers. Two doctors. I told them exactly what to do and they were very willing. That was the craziest thing I've ever done. They met me at a stop sign and they were both really cute. They invited me home and kept following me in this little yellow Mercedes. So in the end, I agreed and told them I'd go with them for just one drink. They took me back to their house and gave me strawberries and champagne. They sat me down

198

in the middle of this huge bed and told me they'd do anything I wanted. That made me feel very horny. So I told them what I wanted and we were screwing all night long.

'The next morning they brought me breakfast in bed on a silver tray with champagne and red roses and asked me to move in with them! I got the hell out of there. They were very nice, but those guys could have slit my throat!'

Model girl Cathy told me of her wonderful night of lust with two men: 'I don't know what came over me that night. I went out to a club, met two blokes, couldn't decide which one I fancied the most, I thought what the hell, and took them both home! For a night of non-stop suck and fuck, you can't beat it. I was sucking one while the other was fucking me, then we swopped around. One guy was fucking me until he'd come and then I'd feel him slip out, and the other guy slap his cock hard inside me. You know those wonderful times, when you're so involved in sex that you completely lose control and it just becomes one big dream. You know, you open your eyes and you don't know where you are, you just know you're getting fucked! It was just like that. Funny thing was that after that crazy night, I started going out with one of the blokes and got quite serious with him. We never mentioned that night, never referred to it or anything, because I was embarrassed that I behaved so much like an animal!'

Here's a wonderfully explicit letter from Dee, a secretary from Croydon who also picked up two men for sex:

I'm blonde, quite pretty with a good figure, and at the grand old age of twenty-four there are obviously some sexual avenues still awaiting my exploration. One particular sexual game that I was desperate to play was the concept of taking on, servicing, being fucked by, call it what you will, two men at one time. The idea of savouring two cocks at once makes my mouth water. One fat greedy dick slipped between the lips of my juicy cunt while another thrusts in and out of my mouth is my fantasy. I could just imagine the sensation; my tongue sliding up and down a bone-hard shaft, while delicately squeezing those bouncing hairy balls, all the while being on all fours, firm hands gripping on to my rounded arse cheeks as a red-hot dick slams into my twitching pussy. The sheer thought of it makes me juice up immediately, as you've probably already ascertained! Just last week I managed to fulfil that fantasy.

One of the girls in the office was leaving, so an after-work drinks do was arranged in a local wine bar. There were about thirty of us from the office, mainly girls, and we ordered lots of wine and set about the process of a piss-up and a good time. Dressed in a cool white suit adorned with golden buttons and featuring a tight skirt that stopped short about three to four inches above the knee, I parked myself on a bar stool and got chatting to two girlfriends.

Some time during the early evening we were joined at the bar by two guys dressed in dark business suits. I found both John and Chris very appealing. John stands about six feet tall, has short dark hair cut close to his head, soulful brown eyes and a wicked lop-sided smile. His buddy Chris is blonde. He has long, flyaway hair, big blue eyes and pearly white teeth. He's a little shorter than his mate, about five eight, or nine, and looks as if he works out. Something clicked in my brain when we got talking. The conversation was rife with sexual innuendo and the atmosphere oozed sensuality. My two friends faded from my attention as I familiarised myself with these attractive men.

By the time the three of us had downed a bottle of champagne, I was ready to leave with them, eager to take them back home to my flat. I knew what I was doing was perhaps not very sensible, but I wanted them both, I wanted them so badly that my pussy ached.

John drove, Chris sat in the back while I rode in the passenger seat up front. As we travelled along the Brighton Road, Chris reached forward and started to massage my neck. I relaxed and slumped down a little in my seat. I felt a tentative hand brush against my inner thigh. Giving John the green light, I spread my legs and wriggled the hem of my skirt brazenly up around my hips. My white knickers were already damp as John started to stroke me through the sheer material. I could feel Chris nibbling on my ear, his hot breath upon my neck.

'Stick it in me!' I squealed as the fabric of my panties was drawn aside and fingers sank into me. With two fingers buried inside my wet slit, John manoeuvered the car expertly, frigging me vigorously, all the time his thumb working my clit. I closed my eyes and screamed in ecstasy: 'Stroke my clit. Ooh, just like that! Oooh, I'm going to come, I'm going to come!' My eyes tightly closed, I unbuttoned my bolero suit jacket, enabling me to play with my nipples through my lacy bra. I squeezed my breasts hard as burning fire exploded in my quivering cunt and I shuddered to a euphoric climax.

Somehow or other we made it home safely. I brushed down my skirt and led the two men through the garden gate, all the while experiencing the warmth of the juices that trickled down my legs. As I put my key in the door John stated in a strident tone: 'You are going to get well and truly fucked, young lady!'

I reached over and, stroking the massive lump in his pants I grinned at both men like a cat who had got all the cream and whispered: 'I do hope so!'

The threesome was all I could ever hope for! Once inside my flat, they stripped me quickly, warm hands and soft fingers caressed me all over. The prospect of two dicks inside my mouth made me tremble with anticipation. Once both John and Chris were unbelted and unzipped, I held a cock in each hand. Alternating my greedy lips from left to right, I sucked first on one and then the other. I was able to get quite a good rhythm going as I stroked them simultaneously, my slithery tongue ever active, my mouth feasting on their knobs. Between mouthfuls I uttered in an urgent whisper: 'I want you both to spunk on my face. I want to feel all that hot come spurting in my mouth, dribbling down my chin.'

Only a few seconds later my desire was fulfilled. John let out a full-throated cry as he shot his creamy load right down the back of my throat. I gagged before swallowing every last drop.

'Suck me, suck me!' grunted Chris as his sperm bubbled up out of his dick all over my face and oozed down my chin to splash on my pink budded breasts. I felt four warm hands reach down to finger my swollen nipples. Pushed back on the sofa, my legs thrust back by my ears, I now enjoyed the sensation of two tongues surrounding my clitoris.

'Taste me. Lick it!' I gasped, my voice thick with sexual excitement. As they slobbered over my cunt, I squashed my heavy tits together. My nipples throbbed and felt like bullets between my fingertips as my whole body started to spasm.

'Oh, I'm coming, I'm coming!' I squealed as they lapped faster and faster, drinking my juices.

A few mintues to compose myself and I was ready for the *pièce de resistance*. I bent over one arm of the sofa and Chris stood before me, thrusting at my face, his engorged cock still slippery from spunk and saliva. My full lips swallowed it all up, taking him deep into my mouth. My back was arched, my arse thrust in the air, and not only was I ready to indulge in a little cocksucking, I was ready to be fucked. By this point in the proceedings I was so horny I would have begged and pleaded to be fucked.

However, that wasn't necessary. I could feel the tip of John's cock as it nuzzled the lips of my pussy. Holding his cock John teased my hot slit with it, gently rubbing it all over my pussy. With Chris still pumping away in my mouth, I reached between my legs and, opening my wet lips wide, I guided John's beautiful rock-hard prick inside my pulsating pussy, the first sensation of penetration sending shivers throughout my entire body and encouraging me to gobble with more enthusiasm on Chris's cock. The whole experience of controlling these two virile men, their two cocks filling up my mouth and cunt, was a little too much for all of us.

Within a few minutes I released Chris from my mouth, his spunk splattering on my face as I once again felt my climax bubbling under the surface. This time I started coming like never before. My orgasm was so intense that it started at my toes and rippled through my body, manifesting its exquisite delights in my throbbing cunt. I felt a hot gush of spunk fill me up, my knees turned weak, and my tongue was a blur on a big red knob, although at this stage in my frenzied passion, I hardly remembered to whom it belonged.

That was the first time. Then Chris politely put forward the proposition that I straddle him and impale myself on his fat cock while his mate sucked on my jiggling breasts, a suggestion that proved amenable to all three participants. Great stuff! Then came the time for some interesting oral play before both men were ready, willing, and able to fuck me again and again and again!

One sex act that fascinates me greatly and wasn't mentioned by any of the women is double penetration, that unbelievable, yet incredible vision that I've seen on screen in many American hard-core movies, when a girl is the recipient of a cock in both her arse and her pussy. I'm not sure I'll ever get round to trying it, but I am very curious to know how it feels!

Porno star Bionca, famous for her anal, orgy and double-penetration scenes in Bruce Seven movies, was obviously the girl to ask. She told me: 'The first sex scene I ever did in front of a camera was an eleven-people orgy, so that was a hell of a way to start! When Bruce makes a movie, the orgy sequence is always the last one to be shot, so it's actually more like a party. Like whatever you want to do, go for it. And we do! Usually we start before the camera starts rolling. I did my first double-penetration scene in a movie called *Loose Ends 2*. Actually it's much better than just doing anal. Double penetration is much better because having a cock in your pussy and your arse at the same time is a great feeling. I don't come when I have anal sex, but I do when I have a dick up my arse and in my pussy. It's very difficult to describe what it feels like, but it makes you feel real hot, especially if you've got another dick in your mouth and a vibrator or a tongue on your clit!'

All of this might be exploring realms that are generally outside the experience of most of us, but it's a mindblowing thought nevertheless! Let's move swiftly on from the delights of double penetration, group sex, orgies, troilism, swapping, swinging, gang-bang parties and any other sexual activity that involves numerous partners, and peruse the next chapter, which will point you in the right direction of the perfect partner – or, if you prefer, perfect partners!

LET'S RECAP!

- 'Many swingers feel that swapping partners brings them closer together. Once you've seen your husband or wife screwing another person, you have shared that emotion, and there is no need to keep secrets any more.'

- 'About thirty men queued up across the dance floor to be serviced by a stunning blonde dressed only in a leather bodice. She went down on her knees and sucked and wanked every one of them off, one by one.'

- 'I realised all of a sudden that the fingers probing my pussy possessed talon-like fingernails. I opened my eyes, glanced towards the stepladder to see a beautiful young woman stroking and fingering my pussy.'

- 'The thing I couldn't cope with was when he was about to fuck her. I just watched his prick penetrate her for the first time and I shouted 'No!' at the top of my voice. I couldn't bear it.'

- 'Threesomes involving two women can finish up with the two females making love to each other while the man droops disappointedly!'

- 'Once both John and Chris were unbelted and unzipped, I held a cock in each hand. Alternating my greedy lips from left to right, I sucked first on one and then the other.'

15

Finding Your Perfect Partner

A recent report on LBC radio revealed research findings from a group of Dutch psychologists who concluded that women appraise a man for only forty-five seconds before deciding whether or not she's found her Mr Right. According to the Eurodocs, in just three-quarters of a minute she will glance firstly at his eyes, then study his hands, paying particular attention to the possibility of a wedding ring adorning the third finger of his left hand, before scrutinising his hair, then his clothes and finally observing his movements and body language. It sounds ludicrous to me that psychologists consider women so fickle that they could come to that decision without the prospective perfect partner uttering one single word!

Funny thing though, love. One woman telephoned the radio station directly after the news item and told the radio presenter and all the station's listeners that the realisation that she had found her perfect partner had hit her in three seconds flat. From just a swift profile glance she was so smitten by the tall, dark, handsome stranger at work that she promptly broke off her engagement with another, and within months had married her Mr Right. The marriage has lasted over forty years, so she must have been a good judge!

I'm not too convinced that love at first sight really

exists. Lust at first sight is quite a different matter, however. How many times have you personally experienced lascivious eye contact across a crowded room, or a fleeting glance stirred a burning desire within to get your greedy hands on that alluring woman or good-looking man? No doubt that sexy scenario has happened to us all at one time or another. It can, of course, progress in several different ways. You could be too shy to make contact and so waste the entire evening hoping that the attractive stranger will save you the embarrassment. Unfortunately they never do! Or, alternatively, you could be just about to make your move and their lover returns with fresh drinks or from a visit to the powder room. If you do sidle over to this luscious sexpot, be they male or female, you may discover they are not quite so appealing close up, or that their personality rubs you up the wrong way immediately and you are forced to beat a hasty retreat before it goes any further. But even worse is the humiliating occasion when you've homed in on your prey and you believe that you're getting on like a house on fire, when he or she disappears to the loo never to return, leaving you feeling high and dry!

But if you're damn lucky, you'll get together and unearth a mindblowing intensity of sensual feeling. On the rare occasions when this happens you'll be on cloud nine, walking in the wondrous sensation of lust at first sight. I don't think there's anything in the world like that moment of sheer bliss when the person you desire makes it apparent that they want you, and that fiery emotion of lust is substantiated and reciprocated. The sex that follows is definitely going to be scorching!

Dierdre, a friend of mine, told me a tale of lust at first sight: 'Michael was one of those men who unleashed an insatiable animal-like passion in me. Every single time I laid eyes on him I wanted to unzip his flies, whip out his cock and feel it probing between the folds of my pink, wet pussy. Michael caused me no end of problems, though, the idyllic situation of carnal lust for each other being blighted only by the fact that we worked closely together. We even had our first fuck in a stationery cupboard during a tea break. Michael just pulled me inside with him, clamped his lips to mine and soon had my soaking panties round my ankles. However, this was not a situation that could continue. I take my job very seriously and was probably in grave danger of being given the sack if fate hadn't intervened. Michael, my fabulous lover, got transferred to Scotland and is no doubt poking his pleasure-filled tool between the cheeks of some other lucky legal secretary as he bends her over his accounting system. So that was the end of a beautiful friendship!'

Lust at first sight is great, but it often doesn't last. So we endure the whole process over and over again in search of our perfect partner. As you've probably surmised, I'm not the kind of woman who thinks a man should always make the first move. Oh no, women are just as entitled to set off in hot pursuit of a little of what they fancy! I know we girls often like to be chased and seduced by men, but sometimes that's not the way things work out. Some extremely eligible men have an extraordinary lack of self-confidence, and in a sense that's part of their appeal. Some females adore pushy, over-confident men, while others love the little boy lost. Personally, I've a penchant for both!

'There's nowt so queer as folk.' When it comes to personal relationships this quaint Northern phrase springs readily to mind. A man is flattered by a woman who is always at his beck and call, and is fascinated by a woman who plays hard to get. You've got to work out how you want to play it, girls and boys! And girls, if you flirt outrageously with him and thrust your

38 DDs under his nose, don't be miffed if he fondles your bottom and suggest you slink off somewhere quiet for a quick fuck! I would advise you start off a little more subtly by being friendly and tactile; touch his hair, brush his fingertips with yours as he hands you a drink. Build up to that moment when you nuzzle your body against his! And don't worry if you succumb to his erotic appeal on your first date. My longest-standing relationship with a lover started off with a frantic fucking session on my living-room floor the very first night we met!

The mating game is something of a big charade, but if you aim to find your perfect partner you are unwittingly forced to become a participant in that game. Of all the billions of people in the world, you are going to come into contact with only a few thousand of them in your lifetime. I'm not suggesting a few thousand as a figure for prospective lovers — that figure refers to *all* the people we may meet during our life, be it at work, at play, or through other means. We may have only a handful of sexual relationships in our lifetime, so it is important that we don't waste time on no-hopers. If it isn't working, move on. Often people cling to disastrous relationships because they are afraid to be alone. That only leads to more trauma in the long run.

In a perfect world I suppose we're all looking for a partner who is not only good looking, charming, generous, amusing, unmarried, and a wonderful lover, but is also stinking rich! Realistically we probably will have to settle for a little less on good looks and filthy lucre, but most of the other attributes can be improved! A word of warning, though — don't try to transform your new partner into something they're not. Trying to change a person to suit your tastes is selfish, and doesn't work. Adjusting to accommodate your partner's likes and dislikes is what it's all about. Plenty of give-and-take and you could be well on the way.

And what about the delicate subject of affairs with a married woman or man? Even a prospective prime minister has recently admitted to an extramarital 'brief relationship'. I'm not going to be a hypocrite and lecture you on the subject. It's obviously not a perfect partnership for the unmarried participant, unless the situation is likely to change, but it can and does work for the ones who can cope. Just be aware of the pain and heartache if you can't handle it!

A colleague of mine conducted a survey amongst friends and acquaintances, asking them to describe their ideal lover. She was shocked to learn that the fantasy figures they described bore little resemblance to their present long-standing partners! It just goes to show that lust at first sight makes for scorching sex in the loo, down a dark alleyway or in the stationery cupboard, but a long-term relationship depends far more on personality that on lust. And how about those couples that we all know that are just so perfectly suited because they're both so irritating or annoying no one else would put up with them? Simply made for each other!

I can't begin to advise you on the perfect pick-up technique because what works for one will probably not work for another. Neither can I tell you where all these rich eligible bachelors and stunningly sophisticated spinsters hang out, but what I can tell you is that you mustn't take it all too seriously. Locating your perfect partner is extremely important, but it's probably going to be a long hard road, and you might as well have some fun along the way!

LET'S RECAP!

- 'That moment of sheet bliss when the person you desire makes it apparent that they want you, and that fiery emotion of lust is substantiated and reciprocated.'

- 'Every single time I laid eyes on him I wanted to unzip his flies, whip out his cock and feel it probing between the folds of my pink, wet pussy.'

- 'We had our first fuck during a tea break in a stationery cupboard. Michael just pulled me inside with him, clamped his lips to mine and soon had my soaking panties around my ankles.'

- 'If you flirt outrageously with him and thrust your 38 DDs under his nose, don't be miffed if he fondles your bottom and suggests you slink off somewhere for a quick fuck.'

- 'In a perfect world I suppose we're all looking for a partner who is not only good looking, charming, generous, amusing, unmarried and a wonderful lover, but is also stinking rich!'

- 'Lust at first sight makes for scorching sex in the loo, down a dark alleyway or in the stationery cupboard.'

16

Sexercises

In the early part of my modelling career I was booked by *Escort* magazine to pose as a gym mistress and perform a series of 'sexercises'. My recollection of the photo session is somewhat vague except I have a clear recall of struggling with a Bullworker and almost having a nasty accident! That fake fitness routine was created for titillation. The exercises I propose in this chapter might well titillate, but they will also ensure that you are in tiptop condition, ready for some vigorous, energetic, immensely enjoyable sex!

There are almost six hundred muscles in the body and all need regular use to keep them working efficiently. Regular exercise raises the metabolic rate so that the cells of the body burn more oxygen. It also improves the condition of the heart, lungs and blood circulation, and eases stress. To maintain fitness you need to exercise for thirty minutes at least three times a week. And in addition to these exercise workouts, many everyday enjoyable activities burn off calories. For instance, dancing the night away at your local nightclub burns up around four hundred and twenty calories an hour and stroking your lover's pleasure zones in an hour of prolonged foreplay can use up approximately one hundred and fifty calories! Sexual intercourse can involve strenuous activity — the energy

213

used in one steamy session can be equivalent to running a two-hundred-metre sprint. It should be obvious that you will enjoy sex all the more if you're basically fit. If you're out of condition and wheezing for breath, that wondrous orgasm is not going to feel quite so good, and I must confess I have a healthy disregard for men who nod off immediately after ejaculation! To be good in bed you need stamina and strength, a robust pelvis, strong arms and legs, and a healthy dose of self-esteem. Once you're confident about your body, whether you've firmed up with exercise or have just learned to love yourself a lttle more, your sex life is bound to improve.

EXERCISES FOR HER

The vagina is made up of a ring of muscles with which the female can grip her lover's cock. These muscles stimulate the penis while making love. Men like a nice tight pussy and there are several ways to keep yours in trim, girls. These simple exercies can make all the difference and enable you to give the man in your life a delightful squeeze just at the right time.

VAGINAL MUSCLES. EXERCISE 1
Wherever you are, whatever you're doing, you can work on tightening your pussy muscles. To contract these muscles just imagine you are bursting for a pee and then squeeze to stop the flow of fluid. This is the contraction of your vaginal muscles and if you spend about a half an hour a day tensing and relaxing these muscles, you'll soon develop a thrilling little twitch.

VAGINAL MUSCLES. EXERCISE 2
Once you've spent a couple of weeks on exercise 1

and your muscles are in good shape, you can practise with a solid object. A dildo, a banana or a cucumber will do. Insert your new friend into your tight pussy, then, using your muscles alone, squeeze it right out of you.

You'd be amazed how strong these muscles can become. I spent several happy holidays in bawdy Bangkok where Oriental girls put on live stage shows to exhibit their unbelievably powerful muscles. I've seen them smoke entire cigarettes, crack eggs and take the tops off Coke bottles just by the use of their vaginal muscles! I'm not expecting you to develop your abilities to the extent that you become some sort of lewd circus act, girls, but remember, your tunnel of love is probably the most exciting area of contact for your man. With your pussy you can caress him, arouse him, control him and eventually bring him to orgasm. That is why it is important to work on those muscles and learn to use them sensitively and effectively.

BREAST EXERCISES
Look after your breasts, girls, and the men in your life will want to look after them too. Neglect them and they may sag. Exercise is the most effective means of improvement. Swimming two or three times a week develops supportive pectoral muscles. And try do-it-yourself hydrotherapy. Spray your breasts daily, firstly with warm water for thirty seconds, then with cold. This will stimulate the blood flow and tighten up the skin.

A word of warning before you start exercising till you drop. A friend of mine started his fitness workout with fifty sit-ups and fifty press-ups and could hardly walk the following day! Start off slowly.

EXERCISES FOR HIM

The most common exercises for men are indeed the most effective.

SIT-UPS
Lie on your back on the floor. Cross your hands beneath the back of your head and sit up without using your hands, and keeping your legs straight out on the floor. Tuck your head tight down towards your groin. Repeat twenty times. This exercise tightens the tummy muscles and strengthens the pelvis.

PRESS-UPS
Lie on the floor face down and, supporting all your weight on your elbows and flats of your hands, raise yourself up and down. Repeat twenty times. This is very good practice for prolonged penetration in the missionary position, chaps!

You should be able to build up to fifty of each of these two exercises a day within a couple of weeks or so.

GENERAL EXERCISES FOR HER TO HELP IMPROVE STAMINA

1. Lie on your back on the floor and lift your buttocks clear of the carpet by supporting your hips with your hands. Hoist your legs in the air and cycle slowly for around twenty-five cycles.
2. Lie on your back on the floor, then sit up without help from your hands and arms. Lean forward and touch your toes. Repeat ten times.
3. Stand with your legs together and hands on hips. Keeping your spine vertical, squat down slowly, then slowly stand up again. Repeat ten times.

With these three exercises you should be able steadily to increase the amount to suit you. These final two exercises are especially for the bum — to keep your rear in gear!

4. Lie on your stomach with your arms by your sides and feet together. Lift one leg as high as you can, cross it over the other leg and touch the floor with your big toe. Alternate with your other leg. Repeat ten times with each leg.
5. Sitting on a chair, hold the sides of the seat, pull in your stomach and your bottom muscles, curl up the pelvis and lift slightly off the chair. Hold for five seconds. Repeat ten times.

And if the thought of all this exercising chills you to the bone, but you really do want to be sexy and fit in bed, here are some fun exercises that you can do at home in the warmth and privacy of your own bathroom. Try Bathercises!

BATHERCISES

FOR THE THIGHS, CALVES AND BOTTOM
Before you get in the bath, stand on the bath mat, feet and legs together, and towel your back and upper body. Cross your ankles. Press legs and calves hard against each other and squeeze, holding for a slow count of six. Release slowly and repeat ten times.

FOR THE CHEST AND SHOULDER MUSCLES
Lie back comfortably in the bath, your head resting on a small, folded-up towel. With your arms at your sides, raise your forearms to a ninety-degree angle in front of you. Keeping shoulders well down, move forearms out sideways, so they rest flat against the sides

of the bath. Push hard against the bath and count to seven. Repeat ten times.

FOR FOOT ARCHES AND CALF MUSCLES

Lie in the same position as for the last exercise. Inch down the bath until your feet are flat against the far end. Push yourself back by pushing away with the balls of your feet, and feel those foot arches and calves flexing. Relax, then repeat fifteen times.

Like all exercises, these will help only if you keep at them and maintain a sensible diet. Additionally, you can improve your fitness by using your initiative. Climb the stairs instead of using a lift whenever possible. Don't drive the car if you only have to travel a half mile or so to the shops — walk or cycle instead. And, dare I say it, if you really don't want to be out of breath when you're making love, why not try cutting down on the cigarettes?

17

Fifty Ways to Please Your Lover

Just to keep that essential variety in your sex life, here's fifty ways to please your lover that should keep you going (perhaps that should be coming?) if you run out of ideas!

1. Let him/her watch you masturbate to orgasm at close proximity.
2. Put on some sexy music, get dressed up in your glad rags and perform a private striptease for your lover.
3. Wake your partner in the middle of the night and perform fellatio or cunnilingus.
4. When he comes home from work, surprise him by greeting him in sexy undies and your spikiest high heels.
5. When she comes home from work, surprise her by greeting her with a whopping great erection!
6. Shave off all your pubic hair.
7. Buy a Polaroid camera and take rude pictues of her sucking you off, or him licking your pussy, or whilst you are actually fucking.
8. Open his flies, or slide your hand into her knickers and play around while he/she is watching their favourite TV show.

9. Ring him/her in the office and talk dirty.
10. Write a raunchy letter to your lover. Explain in graphic detail your dirtiest desires. Use the most explicit, rudest words you can think of.
11. Ask your lover to buy you any item of clothing that they'd like to see you wear for sex, and promise to dress up in it to arouse them.
12. Buy her a strap-on clitoris vibrator and get her to wear it to work.
13. Synchronise your watches and decide upon a time for wicked thought and mutual masturbation while separated from each other.
14. Go to see an erotic movie and play with each other in the back row.
15. Don't let him/her leave for work until you fuck one more time.
16. Turn up at his workplace dressed in a full-length coat, high heels and nothing else. Give him a nice flash when the coast is clear.
17. Go out on the town together, then halfway through the evening whisper in his ear that you've forgotten your panties.
18. Play sex slave for the evening. Your lover's wish is your command.
19. Masturbate together and whoever comes first wins a prize.
20. Try and see if you can deep throat him.
21. Practise oral sex on your lover while he/she is on the telephone to their boss.
22. Challenge him to try to make you come just by kissing and playing with your breasts.
23. Rub several different fruits over your vaginal lips and get him to guess the flavour. Don't let him fuck you unless he guesses correctly.
24. See how far you can stick your tongue up her/his arse.

25. Ask him to ejaculate over a different part of your body each time you make love.

26. Ask him/her to reveal their most decadent sex fantasy, and if it's possible, act it out!

27. Masturbate him with whipped cream, strawberry yogurt or something equally gooey and messy.

28. Slide a ripe strawberry inside your cunt and ask him to eat it out.

29. Make love in the most outrageous spot you can think of — in a lift, or a in a graveyard.

30. Try out a new sexual position every night of the week.

31. Dress up in his favourite uniform and indulge in a little role-playing.

32. Tell an erotic story, each taking a turn as the steamy saga progresses.

33. Buy an erotic magazine and read each other dirty letters.

34. Ask to watch him/her pee.

35. Ask him/her to wash you in the bath or shower.

36. Walk around your home naked all day long.

37. On a summer's afternoon, drive out into the country and make love on the grass.

38. Drive out to a secluded spot and have a quickie fuck in the back seat of the car.

39. List all the places in your home that are possible locations for sex. Then fuck your way around the house.

40. Massage each other with your favourite scented oils.

41. Serve him dinner wearing thigh-length boots and erotic nipple jewellery.

42. Ask him to spank you.

43. Slip a sexually explicit photo of yourself into your lover's pocket and let him/her discover it at work.

44. Tie him to the bed, sit on his face and tease him

unmercifully. Only let him fuck you when you are good and ready.

45. Play with your lover whenever you get the chance — in the back of a taxi, or in a restaurant.

46. Play at being a glamour model. Dress up in your favourite undies and pose for him/her.

47. Make her feel expensive with champagne. Dribble the cold liquid over her breasts and suck it from her nipples, then ease the neck of the bottle into her pussy and shake gently for that fizzy feeling!

48. Use your vibrator on his penis, or slide it up his arse.

49. Surprise him by inserting your vibrator up your arse while he's fucking you.

50. Sit on his face and tell him that you love him!

Adopt and adapt any of these sexy suggestions that you feel will suit your personal circumstances and add that extra bit of spice to your love life. Some of my ideas will no doubt tickle your fancy and have the potential to develop into outrageous, unbelievable sex sessions. You may, on the other hand, turn your nose up in disgust at some of them, but if the lady in your life displays a desire to wank you while your dick is a mass of whipped cream, or your man shows a keen interest in watching you urinate, why not allow them their fun? Some of these naughty notions may even have you doubled up with laughter, but the ability to inject a little humour into your lovemaking is also important. Not all of your efforts will be a resounding success, so don't be afraid to laugh with your lover during sex. The most important aspect of these suggestions is that they are designed to make you feel comfortable about your sexuality, to assist you and your lover discuss what kind of sex games to play, and enable you as a couple to explore your likes and dislikes.

I'm not advocating you try out my inventive love ideas daily — your lover might think you're some kind of demented prankster — but every now and again dip into my pleasure guide and select a suggestion that suits you. Whether you're shaving off each other's pubic hair or fingering and fumbling in the back row of the cinema, you can be sure your sex life will improve and never be boring! Each new sex game and challenge won't always be an ecstatic experience, but just by being a participant in the game, it will demonstrate to your lover that you're sexually resourceful, on the ball, and eager to please. Because after all, learning to please is what this book has been all about. I hope you've had as much fun reading it as I've had writing it! Have a happy, healthy, horny sex life!

Love
Luigi